Parish

Parish Nursing
Stories of Service and Care

Verna Benner Carson and
Harold G. Koenig

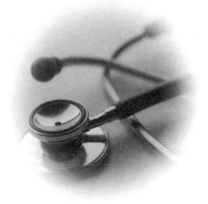

Templeton Foundation Press
Philadelphia & London

Templeton Foundation Press
Five Radnor Corporate Center, Suite 120
100 Matsonford Road
Radnor, Pennsylvania 19087

Designed and typeset by Kachergis Book Design
Printed by Hamilton Printing Company

LIBRARY OF CONGRESS CATALOGING-IN-PUBLICATION DATA

Carson, Verna Benner.
    Parish nursing : stories of service and care / Verna Benner Carson and Harold G. Koenig.
        p.   cm.
    Includes bibliographical references and index.
    ISBN 1-890151-88-2 (alk. paper)
    ISBN 1-890151-94-7 (pbk. : alk. paper)
    1. Parish nursing.   2. Parish nursing—Anecdotes.   3. Pastoral medicine.   I. Koenig, Harold G.   II. Title.
    RT120.P37 C374 2002
    610.73'43—dc21

                                                        2002019157

Printed in the United States of America

02 03 04 05 06 07   10 9 8 7 6 5 4 3 2 1

To my husband John Carson
To my wife Charmin Marie Koenig

Contents

Foreword

Many years ago, when I might have been described as a "wild and crazy guy," I worked as a full-time hospital chaplain and educator, a part-time counselor and family therapist, *and* served as pastor for two small, urban churches. The two churches had more than their share of elders, plus a variety of folks who had lived much of their lives in the projects. Almost everyone in those two churches could have been considered as having unmet health needs.

Having heard Granger Westberg tell of his dream for parish nurses, I went to visit a nurse who was a member of one of the churches I was serving. After I explained Westberg's vision I asked, "Do you think we might do something like that?" Her response was quick and immediate, "Of course we can!" Then she added, "I didn't realize it, but I've been waiting for something like this." That was my first experience with parish nursing.

It is now many, many years later, and this volume is filled with the stories of nurses who have also responded to the call to serve as parish nurses. Responding to that call has never been more crucial than now:

- Despite the ever growing research literature that links religion and participation in religious activity with increased health and decreased morbidity, very few seminaries prepare pastors for this important intersection of health and faith.

- The number of persons over age sixty-five is increasing exponentially but the capacity of the American health-care system to meet these needs has not—and perhaps cannot—kept pace.
- Prevention provides the "biggest bang for the buck" in terms of maintaining a positive health status, but dollars for prevention are among the first to be cut from the budgets of managed-care organizations.
- Making meaning out of life events such as health crises, chronic disability, death, and dying is a central task for hundreds of thousands Americans.

Pastors of local congregations are often bewildered by medical terminology and the inner workings of managed care. Combine this with never-ending demands on their time, and one can see that most pastors are neither equipped nor have time for the ministry of health care.

Professional health-care chaplains, because of their extensive post-graduate education and certification, are well prepared to deal with the specialized setting, language, and demands of modern medicine. However, such chaplains are usually found only in academic medical centers, community hospitals, or long-term care facilities.

Day in and day out, it is the parish nurse—in those congregations fortunate enough to have such a person on the staff—whose job description blends the medical with the spiritual to provide the sort of care both pastors and professional chaplains want for people on a day-to-day basis.

The chapters in this volume relate the stories, tasks, and preparation for the work of the parish nurse. Among the tasks presented (as described by Westberg, Holstrom, and Sensenig) are three I think are especially important: health educator, health counselor, and health advocate. It is not that the others are not important, for they are. These three are of particular importance (from my point of view, at least) because they represent activities of ministry that especially complement the work of pastors who do not—and likely will not—have these skills.

Body-mind-spirit is an increasingly familiar phrase to those of us who have worked for so long to integrate spirituality and health. It is not a subject often taught in seminary. In fact, it may be that a greater percentage of medical and nursing schools (impacted by the generosity of Templeton grants) deal with these issues than do seminaries. Therefore, to have a parish nurse who is a *health educator* to members of congregations regarding the great variety of issues associated with health (blood pressure, smoking, health-risk behaviors, cancer prevention, and so forth) is not only a boon to both pastor and congregation, it is a vital witness to the unity of body, mind, and spirit.

Prevention and education take on an especially personal focus when associated with individuals. There are numerous stories here of women and men whose lives have been impacted for the better because of the *health counselor* role of the parish nurse. Seldom do congregants/parishioners talk with the pastor about their health issues. They will—and do—open up to the parish nurse about these concerns. Assessing depression, referring for a work-up following blood-pressure screening, and counseling regarding diet or smoking are not only appropriate but vital tasks in any congregation that understands the human body as the temple of God.

Whether it is an HMO or other expression of managed care, the medical care system is usually difficult to negotiate. The language is foreign, the procedures are arcane, and rights are a mystery. The parish nurse as *health advocate* is often uniquely prepared and situated to help parishioners/congregants navigate this minefield of potential problems. The relief experienced by people who have such an advocate is palpable.

I need to say one final word about parish nurses. Christians, whether Roman Catholic or Protestant, liberal or conservative, have an increasing sense of the "ministry of the laity." It is in our baptism that each Christian person is called into ministry. A few of us are ordained to particular ministries within congregations such as teaching, preaching, and the celebration of the sacraments. Every one of us, however, has within us the gifts for some ministry to and for God's people.

Parish nurses are called out and equipped in special ways to exercise a ministry of health. Without this ministry the church is the poorer and God's people are less well served. I am honored with this opportunity to introduce this volume about parish nurses, for they are my colleagues in the work of the gospel, and more than once, they have been the ones to re-present the gospel to me in times of need.

LAUREL ARTHUR BURTON, TH.M., TH.D., BCC
Academic Dean and Professor of Pastoral Studies
The Methodist Theological School in Ohio
Past President of the Association of Professional Chaplains
Chairman, The COMISS Network

Preface

Before there were word processors, computers, typewriters, or other implements to write with, there were stories. The collective wisdom of generations has been passed down through storytelling. Stories spark the imagination; they inspire and motivate; they teach and encourage; they correct and challenge. Stories are indeed powerful. And so we have chosen to present the stories of parish nurses—to allow you to hear them describe their journeys in their own voices. Hopefully you will learn from them, be inspired and motivated by them, and allow your imagination free reign to envision parish nursing operating in your church and your health-care system.

We believe that parish nursing offers hope to a beleaguered and increasingly inadequate health-care system where the demands for care, especially long-term care, are outstripping the available resources. There is growing discontent with our medical system. At the same time it is touted to be technologically the best in the world, it is criticized for its neglect of the person. While costs continue to rise, care continues to diminish. Witness the increased interest and involvement in alternative and complementary medical practices such as herbology, acupuncture and acupressure, therapeutic touch, crystal therapy, and reflexology just to name a few. Certainly this trend can be partially explained by the dissatisfaction people feel toward traditional medicine. People want to be cared for in a wholistic manner—to be heard, to share in decision making about their lives, to be loved even when they are unlovable, to be accepted as they are in their brokenness, to be encouraged to delineate their own values, goals, and personal views, and to be recognized as more than a diseased gall bladder or a serious case of depression. Patients want health-care providers to see beyond presenting symptoms to the impact of these symptoms on their lives, their work, their capacity to experience joy, their ability to engage in family life, and their experience of spirituality. Patients have always known that they are so much more than the divisible components of body and mind that are the focus of most medical treatment. In truth, real care recognizes that people are indivisible wholes—fully integrated physical, emotional, intellectual, social, and spiritual beings. Parish nurses recognize this and respond to it.

There is an old adage that says that there is really nothing new under the sun—just old ideas rediscovered and repackaged. Whether this adage is generally true or not, it is certainly true for parish nursing with its focus on "caring for" rather than curing. This "new" specialty represents a return to the Judeo-Christian roots of nursing. Jesus focused on the meaning of suffering and the healing of the whole person; he made little distinction between healing of the body, mind, or spirit. There was emphasis on the thought life of the individual to affect health and the power of prayer to affect healing.

Some of the earliest nurses believed that their sole purpose was to honor Christ's commands to minister to the least fortunate among them. They recognized that caring for others extended beyond ministry to physical needs. Their care included providing intellectual and spiritual nourishment, clothing others with human kindness and concern, remembering individuals who had been forgotten or neglected and no longer cared for and loved, and providing hospitality for people who were homeless or who felt lost in a strange environment. In their ministrations, these nurses saw spiritual meaning in the care they extended. They believed that when they cared for the ill and needy in this fashion, they were serving not only the ill, but God.[1]

Over the years, nursing gradually moved away from its spiritual roots. It expanded beyond church-based hospitals and moved into secular institutions of care. Nursing preparation, initially controlled by religious orders, moved into the atmosphere of the state-controlled university setting. The twentieth century saw upheaval in all areas of nursing. Professional organizations were developed to exercise control over nursing practice; educational programs delineated levels of practice and different roles for nurses depending on preparation; licensure came about as a way of ensuring nursing competence; nursing focused increasingly on the scientific and technological advances that were occurring throughout health care and integrated these advances into nursing education and practice. Wholistic care and especially a recognition of the importance of spirituality, faith, and religion to a person's health took a back seat to "high-tech" interventions. For a time, "high-touch" had certainly moved out of fashion with the nursing profession.

However, even with these changes, there always remained a cadre of nurses who kept alive the vision and mission of nursing and held fast to the belief that the essence of nursing is to care about and for the whole person. The theme of service and ministry is evident in the writings of many of the twentieth-century nursing leaders.

As the twentieth century came to a close, there was growing dissatisfaction among nurses regarding the movement of the profession away from a focus on the whole person. Nurses expressed concern that increasingly there was little distinction between nursing and medical care. This discontent among nurses led to the development of organizations such as Nurses' Christian Fellowship and the American Holistic Nurses Association. Both of these organizations focus on the spiritual aspects of health—the former does so from a Christian perspective and publishes the *Journal of Christian Nursing*, and the latter does so from a perspective encompassing other spiritual traditions and publishes the *Journal of Holistic Nursing*.

In the 1980s, the Reverend Granger Westberg "rediscovered" church-based nursing and called it parish nursing. It is in honor of Rev. Westberg that we use the word "wholistic" rather than "holistic." He believed strongly that the "w" was essential to connote the "whole person,"[2] which is the focus of the parish or congregational nurse. This ministry began as one strongly connected and rooted in the Christian faith. However, just as the earliest Christian nursing practice was inclusive rather than exclusive, extending health care to both Christian and non-Christian communities, the concept of parish nursing has spread beyond the Christian church. Even within the *Scope and Standards of Parish Nursing Practice* this specialty is defined as ". . . a unique, specialized practice of professional nursing that focuses on the promotion of health within the context of the values, beliefs, and practices of a faith community, such as a church, synagogue, or mosque and its mission and ministry to its members (families and individuals), and the community it serves."[3]

Recognizing that the focus of parish nursing extends beyond Christian theology, we attempted to identify nurses involved in parish nursing who represent other faith traditions so that we could include their stories. To this end, unfortunately, we were less than successful. We did include the story of Linda Weinberg, a Jewish congregational nurse, who practices in the Philadelphia area. We sought information from leaders within the parish-nurse movement regarding their knowledge and contacts with nurses from non-Christian faith traditions. For instance, Rosemarie Matheus reported that the hospital system with which she is associated in Milwaukee approached an Islamic congregation with a proposal to partner with them in parish nursing. Several years ago Rosemarie spoke to a group of Moslem nurses at an international conference of nursing held in Jordan. There was only mild interest at the time. We "heard" about a parish nurse serving a Buddhist congregation in the Chicago area, another nurse who practices parish nursing in California with the Vedanta Society, a Hindu tradition, and a nurse involved in health ministry for the Unitarian Universalist Church. However, our attempts to connect with these nurses were futile—perhaps, an excellent reason for a sequel!

This book tells the stories of parish nurses as they journey into a territory largely uncharted where the road map, the directions, and the rules of the road are being discovered as they move forward. Their words present stories of hearing God's call, of their responses to this call, of their faith that they are doing the "right thing," of their joys, sorrows, and challenges, and of their quiet determination and dedication as they offer their time and talents to meet the needs of others. Their stories inspired us and we are grateful for the generous spirit of so many nurses. They responded to our questionnaire; they answered countless e-mails; they shared their resources so that we might share them with you; they opened their hearts to us just as they open their hearts to the congregants they serve. We hope that this book honors parish nurses and serves as an encouragement to other nurses to respond to that gentle "God-nudge" they may be feeling. We hope too that the book inspires church members and leaders as well as health-care providers and administrators to explore the values and benefits of parish nursing within their own faith traditions and to the health-care system at large.

Parish Nursing

CHAPTER I

Responding to the Call

 *The watchman opens the door for this man, and the sheep listen to His voice and heed it; and He calls his own sheep by name and brings them out. When he has brought his own sheep outside, he walks on before them, and the sheep follow him because they know his voice. They will never follow a stranger, but will run away from him because they do not know the voice of strangers or recognize their call. I am the Good Shepherd, and I know and recognize my own and My own know and recognize Me. (John 10:3–5,14)*

"Shhh, I think I hear my mom calling." Johnny hushed his friend and inclined his ear toward a distant sound. "Nah, I don't hear nothin'. You must be imaginin' it," his friend said. Laughing, Johnny responded, "That's my mom all right. I know her yell anywhere."

How many of us respond to this scenario? There are voices that we recognize immediately—no one needs to tell us if the voice belongs to a loved one, a friend, an adult, a child, or a stranger. We respond because each voice is unique, just as each person is unique. An unborn baby responds to the voice of her mother, and at birth immediately orients herself to that most familiar and comforting sound of her mother's voice.

Just so each of us hears the voice of God and we decide whether or not to respond to that voice. Unlike other voices that can be demanding, seductive, angry, or threatening, God's call to us, although recognizable, can be ignored and pushed aside. God's voice is loving and gentle, albeit persistent. He calls each of us to serve and honor Him in unique ways—through the many roles we fulfill, chosen vocations and avocations, volunteer activity, quiet time, and relationships.[1] Many times the response to God's call requires not only sacrifice but also faith that God will not abandon us in strange territory. In Genesis we read the story of Abraham, who uprooted his family and left his country and all that was familiar and comfortable in response to God's call and promise to multiply Abraham's descendants and from them create a great nation. Abraham's journey was not easy, but he trusted God and he moved forth.

Likewise nurses hear the call of the Lord—a call to serve Him by caring for His wounded people in hospitals, clinics, homes, shelters, schools, businesses, and church communities.[2] Sometimes the call and the direction desired by God is very clear, other times the call is vague and requires time for the nurse to comprehend fully what God is asking, still other times the call is unsettling and unwanted and the nurse resists responding because to do so requires moving out of a zone of comfort and security.[3] Regardless of how the call is received, increasing numbers of nurses are hearing God calling them out of what is familiar and placing them into virtually new and uncharted territory of church communities. The journey is both exciting and frightening. Karaban states that at the heart of a call to ministry is the story of an encounter between an individual and God.[4] Let's listen to the stories of parish nurses, hear their voices, and experience their encounters with God.

Marianne Parker first served as a volunteer parish nurse before moving into the position of parish nursing program coordinator for St. Joseph's Hospital in Syracuse, New York. Marianne tells her own story:

> AS A NURSING STUDENT I entertained transient thoughts about working on the Good Ship Hope—a floating medical mission. I wasn't interested in this because of a "heart for

mission"; rather, something about traveling from place to place caring for the needy appealed to me. I hadn't attended church since high school. Like so many, I wandered away during the college years. I met my future husband and the gentle call of medical mission was quickly drowned out by a wonderful courtship. I dreamed about becoming a midwife when I graduated from nursing school in 1982, but again, God had a different plan. I married and became a mother instead.

My nursing career took back seat to being a wife and mother and although there were times of frustration, part-time work in cardiac and intensive care fit family needs well . . . until my self-imposed "super-mom/super-nurse" expectations led to burnout, sleep deprivation, and bitterness. It was at this point that I came to know Jesus Christ as my personal Lord and savior. God met me in my "brokenness," healed and reshaped me. Through music and mentors, the Holy Spirit brought to my remembrance many Christian lessons I had learned as a child and walked away from as a young adult. I began writing and singing inspirational and educational songs on a guitar that had been silent for many years. Gradual transformation ensued and continues every day.

God planted me in a church and I began searching for ways to serve and honor Him. God bent down, reached out to me, and called me by name. An overwhelming desire to know Him and serve His people grew and grew. "I" tried many things. I was a Sunday school teacher, library aide, visitor of the sick, and doer of anonymous good deeds, small group leader, and dreamer of dreams. My purpose was clear. Christ was calling me to show and share His love with a broken and needy world, but I didn't know what this call would look like.

I had the compulsion to learn about my church, its diverse ministries, and the people that served in them. I studied spiritual gifts and created a small group Bible study focusing upon spiritual gifts and ministry creation. I created a Gift Ministry Notebook to identify church programs and possible spiritual gifts that would empower the ministries. A small group of women started a mentoring program to match people's gifts, passions, and experience to ministry needs. The timing wasn't right. Support for the ministry faded. I felt that I had failed. A desire to participate in evangelistic outreach uniting all of the Christian congregations in our town took hold. God was pruning and preparing me.

My young family grew and all three children were soon in school full days. I knew this meant I would return to full-time nursing duty. I prayed that God would allow me to work for Him full time. In June of 1997 I shared a "popcorn idea" with my pastor. What if . . . we did health education and screening from the church and made ourselves and Christian information available to those who came? As a stranger to the parish nurse movement, I thought the concept was original. He agreed to explore the idea.

I also began searching for full-time nursing employment at this time. The director of wellness and disease control at the hospital where I was presently employed described a mall-based community wellness program, but it didn't have much appeal because the location was more than twenty miles from my home. "What do you think about . . . starting wholistic wellness programs in churches?" I asked. She replied, "As a matter of fact, we have a brand new position for just that. Maybe you would want to apply." I hung up the phone, raised my hands in praise, and thanked God for my new job. A few weeks after the interview, I got the call about my job. "We've decided to hire someone else." I was devastated, but God is good. One of my close friends, who had arrived five minutes before the call, comforted and cried with me. For a while I doubted my belief that God was actually calling me! However, God's timing is perfect and His plan better than anything we can imagine.

Months later, I met the wellness director in the hospital. She said, "Are you still interested in parish nursing?—because the job is yours if you want it. The previous coordinator has gone back to school." I became St. Joseph's Hospital Parish Nursing Program coordinator in September 1997. I continue to water the seeds planted by the first coordinator, pull out the weeds, and bring in the harvest that God grows.[5]

Carole Kornelis had experienced God's hand in her life for many years, not only in her "reaching out activities" but in her own struggles and eventual healing through those struggles.

HAVING BEEN INVOLVED in teaching and leading groups from kindergarten to twelfth grade, I felt that God eventually would lead me into a ministry that related to my nursing. When the idea of parish nursing was presented as a possibility, I was elated. I knew that this was a God-given opportunity to use my nursing talents on an entirely different level from what I could do in the secular world. I could use the trials and losses I had endured over the past eight years and help others heal from their wounds. I was "free" to be me, a Child of the King![6]

Susan Dyess believes that she received two very distinct calls from God. The first was to be a nurse. The second, to be a parish nurse, was specific and quite different from her lifelong knowledge that God wanted her to enter nursing. She experienced both callings with increasing intensity over a period of time and felt a strong sense that God was always leading her to something more. Her response to God's call, although experienced as "right," also represented something of a departure from where the majority of her nurse colleagues stood. This sense of being separated from the group to stand with and for God in a unique role is a common theme in the stories of the Old Testament prophets. Susan explains:

I FELT DIFFERENT from other nurses because I was trying to live my professional life according to my personal truths. I came to understand that I was a vessel for the Lord to work through. Specific Scripture brought me to an increased awareness of my intended purpose in life. The journey to this realization was not recognized in a moment but rather occurred as a process of realization over several years of personal and professional growth. Truly I sensed a calling to be more than I was capable of. It was a powerful and unfamiliar call. Yet I had a knowing that I was walking with the Lord, and so His peace was present.[7]

Catherine Lomax, a parish nurse at the Church of the Good Samaritan in Paoli, Pennsylvania, had plans to "relax, smell the roses, and otherwise enjoy life" when she heard the Lord's call. Catherine initially experienced the call as a gentle longing or tugging of her heart that over time took on a greater urgency and specificity. She began a two-year journey of personal discovery and spiritual preparation before God's call to parish nursing became clear to her.

TWO YEARS BEFORE taking the parish nursing position, I left my full-time case-management position at Paoli Hospital. I thought to smell the roses, to relax, and to pursue all the things I had wanted to do. God had other ideas for me. In those two years he brought me through a course on boundaries and made me look at what was holding up my life. The issue of forgiveness came out of this introspection. I had difficulty forgiving other people and myself. This discovery was very releasing and I started to move forward in my journey. We went on our second trip to Habitat for Humanity in North Carolina and there in a lowly old tobacco barn I found myself painting shelves for a house we were building. My Lord was waiting in the barn for me and put in my heart that He needed me, for what I did not know. Later while singing Psalm 139, "Search Me and Know Me," in our church choir, I found myself listening intently and feeling the meaning of the words. I ventured forth in response to what I believed was God's call and threw myself into all kinds of service activities. I became a volunteer at a local hospital and signed up for the homeless mission at church—serving became my life. I read a book entitled *Let Prayer Change Your Life* by Becky Tirabassi. I started to keep a journal and dedicated the first hour of the day to this activity. I read and prayed about Scripture. It brought me release and comfort to begin to see the Bible in a clear light. There were things happening in my life that only God through prayer could do. At the end of my two years in my new life of service to Him, He called me to a job called parish nursing, where I could combine my skills as a nurse with His word as I serve His people.[8]

God sometimes uses our pain and neediness to grab our attention and focus our thinking. This was the case for Ellen Altenhofer, who was in the midst of juggling the demands of primary caregiving to her mother; during that time Eileen came face-to-face with the inadequacies of the current health-care system.

DURING 1992, I was the primary caregiver for my mother throughout her terminal illness with cancer and found that accessing community resources was incredibly difficult and frustrating even though I was a nurse. It was almost impossible to get the help that I needed. I thought that if it was hard for me—someone who has an understanding of the health-care system—it must be impossible for lay people in a similar situation. I wondered what could be done to help others suddenly thrust into the role of caregiver. When I asked the home health agency for assistance in obtaining respite care, it was suggested that I contact my church. Shortly after my mother passed away, two opportunities presented themselves—a lay parish caregiving program entitled "Called to Care" and parish nurse training. I literally could not sleep! My thoughts were consumed with the possibilities that lay before me.

In January of 1993 our minister, Terry Teigen, began an extensive training series to prepare us to become lay caregivers. Terry helped us to explore how we would go about developing our caregiving ministry as well as the practical skills relating to visiting and communication. We also focused on specific caregiving situations such as cancer, grief, divorce, and unemployment. The training series culminated with an exploration of "Resource of Faith," which examined the foundations found in prayer and Bible study for a caregiving ministry. Twelve of us completed the training series and began our service to the members of our congregation. Under Terry's direction we formed the Parish Care Committee to determine how to address the needs of the congregation. In the fall of 1994 I became the coordinator of our Parish Care Program. At that time Pacific Lutheran University was offering a course entitled "Introduction to Parish Nursing." The brochure stated that one of the functions of a parish nurse was to coordinate volunteers, so it seemed a perfect opportunity to develop skills to assist me in my leadership of the Called to Care Program.[9]

Pauline Sheehan of Everett, Washington, also heard the Lord's call in the midst of pain and discouragement.

IT WAS A TIME of hospital mergers; one whole floor of the hospital was shut down. Many of the staff were laid off and those who were left lived in constant fear of who would be next. For a while the remaining staff (including me) became critical and depressed—the heart went out of our service to patients. Then out of nowhere God gave me an idea about a role for nurses that combined some of the chaplain's services with those of an RN. I didn't even realize at the time that there was such a thing as a parish nurse![10]

Rose Young believed that she heard clearly the Lord's call to ministry but discovered as she proceeded that she and the Lord sometimes had different plans and timing!

I RECEIVED THE CALL for parish nursing approximately ten years ago when I was still working full time as an instructor of practical nursing. Since that time I have used every spare moment to follow the Lord's leading in that direction. After retiring from working part time as a staff nurse and full time as an instructor, I attended Geneva College to update my counseling M.A. at a college that could include the study of religions as part of the curriculum. I then wrote a proposal for UPMC Horizon Hospital, serving Greenville and Farrell, Pennsylvania, for a parish nursing program based out of the hospital.

For four months I was given the freedom to investigate programs throughout the country; I obtained copies of several programs and I had telephone conversations with several parish nurses. Plans were made to invite ministers and nurses throughout the country to a seminar about parish nursing. We had invited Norma Small, Ph.D., CRNP, who was the Standards of Practice advisor from Johnstown, Pennsylvania and former dean of Georgetown University School of Nursing. I was in "seventh heaven" believing that my dream and calling were being realized. The Lord however was working on a different schedule than mine! The day before the invitations were to be mailed I received a call from the director of Community Outreach with whom I had been working. I was told to halt the plans for the program. I was so disappointed—but actually not too surprised. I had sensed for some time that he was viewing the program more as a marketing technique for the hospital than as a service. Since another hospital had heard that we were doing this seminar they were making similar plans. Now the director of Community Outreach wanted to take our hospital in another direction to meet the community's needs. In spite of this setback I continued with efforts to arrange a meeting at my church (on a much smaller scale) and invited three other parish nurses from the area to serve on a panel. I told Joy Conti and Norma Small, nurses who had been very helpful in the past, of my plans to have regular meetings to inform other nurses about parish nursing and include speakers from various services in the community. This was in the fall of 1998. That same year my church council voted to accept me officially as their parish nurse.[11]

The Old Testament is replete with stories of how God spoke to His people through dreams. Joseph knew through a dream that he would rise up above his brothers and that they would reverence him (Genesis 37:5–9). God also gave Joseph the ability to interpret dreams and through this gift Joseph was able to foretell Egypt's future for Pharaoh. Pharaoh rewarded Joseph for his gift by giving him authority over all of Egypt (Genesis 40 and 41). In the New Testament, another Joseph, betrothed to Mary, had a dream in which an angel gave Joseph a message from God. Joseph was told that rather than quietly abandoning the pregnant Mary, he was to take her as his wife. Joseph was obedient to God. He married Mary and raised Mary's baby as his own. He thus fulfilled his part in bringing to pass the Scripture passage foretelling that a virgin would become pregnant and give birth to a son—the son of course was Jesus (Matthew 1:20–24)! Today God's messages may seem less dramatic than those received by Joseph of the Old Testament and Joseph of the New Testament. However, God still speaks to people through dreams. Let's look at Barb McDonald's dream and how this dream came true. With the support and encouragement of her pastor, Barb presented the following to her congregation.

> I HAVE A DREAM. I have had a dream for a long time—one that I hope you will share with me. I see a need in our church, our community for a helping hands group—the "Dream Team"! This would include such things as doing yard work for the elderly or ill or those who just can't do for themselves. Perhaps working inside the home to paint, wash windows, do minor repairs such as plumbing, etc. Perhaps small car repairs, whatever your talent

might be. Someone to visit the ill or elderly or shut-ins—to take a plate of cookies or just a smile and a cheery "hello," to play a game or read a book. Perhaps to stay with a family member while the caregiver goes out for a while. To do this we need help: a few people to form a committee to put this together; a list of people willing to help and to share their talents; and most of all a list of people who need something done. I see this as a way of sharing the talents God has given us, of sharing God's love with those around us, of taking God's love out to the community. If this is your dream or if you are willing to share mine you can see me after church to talk about it, or give me a call. I would love to hear from you.[12]

This is how Barb started the "Dream Team," which became the foundation for a parish nurse ministry. It didn't take long to develop that list of people willing to share their time and talents. It actually took much longer to discover who actually needed the help! Barb believes that it is difficult for many people to admit that they need help and many times the expressed need came through a referral. Her move into the position of parish nurse seemed a natural progression from "Dream Team" work—she had organized a volunteer network, one of the key roles for the parish nurse!

Sometimes the Lord calls nurses to be "the" parish nurse for a congregation. But just as God's kingdom has many mansions, within parish nursing there are many roles—all necessary, all equally important. Ann Solari-Twadell, a recognized leader in the parish nurse movement, has a different story to tell as she responded to God's calling to set up a centralized resource for nurses interested in parish nursing.

IN 1986, I was the Director of Nursing for the Specialty Hospital for Addiction Treatment of Lutheran General Health System. The financing for addiction treatment was slowly being eliminated. Knowing this I went to my supervisor, Reverend

John Keller, and talked about leaving my current position. . . . I did not want to leave Lutheran General, for I liked their institutional philosophy of Human Ecology.

Reverend Keller suggested that I talk with Reverend James Wiley, the Vice President of Church Relations at Lutheran General. I did so, and this resulted in my working on a pilot project called Congregational Health Partnership. I can remember sitting in my office after leaving the Director of Nursing position [and] wondering what is this all about? How does this work fit? All I could do was trust that God had something important in mind.

At the same time, the parish nurse program was being piloted at Lutheran General Hospital. The six parish nurses were trying to figure out their roles and pioneer the beginnings of parish nursing. . . . Granger Westberg was making his way around the country talking about this new concept of "parish nursing." The problem was that as people became excited, Granger would leave town. These excited folks would try to contact the six nurses in the six churches to find out how this was done. The part-time nurses had little time to consult with others. I went to my supervisor and suggested the concept of a parish nurse resource center. It was endorsed and in 1986 the work began.[13]

Up until October 2001, the International Parish Nurse Resource Center was a major force in the evolving growth and structure of parish nursing not only across the United States, but in Canada, Korea, and Australia. The International Parish Nurse Resource Center was responsible for developing the standardized Basic Parish Nurse Curriculum and the Basic Parish Nurse Coordinator/Manager Curriculum that is widely used for the preparation of parish nurses and parish nurse leaders. The International Parish Nurse Resource Center also convened annual educational programs where nurses met to learn about current parish nurse activities; provided consultants to churches, hospitals, agencies, and religious denominations interested in organizing parish nursing in their institutions; and published many resources for the growth of parish nurses including a quarterly publication titled *Perspectives in Parish Nursing Practice,* published by Advocate Health Care and edited by Ann Solari-Twadell.

Rosemarie Matheus, the director of the Parish Nurse Preparation Institute at Marquette University College of Nursing, tells her story of responding to God's call. Similarly to Ann Solari-Twadell, Rosemarie was not called to *become* a parish nurse but to use her teaching skills to develop a curriculum for parish nurses.

DURING ONE OF MY early nursing classes the instructor directed us to write five- and ten-year goals for ourselves. I tried . . . but I couldn't. Life didn't present itself to me as if I was in control. I wasn't able to convince the instructor (who much later was a student in one of my parish nurse classes) that this wasn't the way I saw my future . . . all organized and planned. What about the plan God had for me, which at that time I was just beginning to understand? What was I to do with all the unexpected, unknown opportunities that were ahead and didn't get written into my five- and ten-year goals? What was I to do with them? Today, I am more convinced that I was right, for I have never had the daring to write long-term goals. God has brought me to places I would never have imagined, let alone committed to paper. It was if God was speaking to me the words he spoke to Jeremiah, "Call unto me, and I will show you great and mighty things, which you know not."

I was an only child, a "latch-key child" before the term was coined. Families seemed like a fantasy that other people were part of. I didn't plan to have five children . . . but God again had a ten-year plan for me. Two girls and three boys in ten years. Along with their spouses (my pseudo children) they have brought six grandchildren into my still-growing family. Nursing had to wait until I had given my all in the nurturing of these "gifts" from God. Then His call came back to me; I was to again use the talents He had given me for nursing. While my children were in high school and college, I too was in college getting my bachelor's and then my master's degree in pediatrics . . . what else, I had all the practical experience not only from my own children who taught me volumes, but from my professional experience working at a juvenile prison for boys. Upon finishing my degrees, I again thought perhaps I should have a written goal, but before I could force myself to create one, God's master plan stepped in.

Three months after graduating from Marquette University College of Nursing with my new degree in teaching and pediatrics, I was asked to join the faculty and teach sophomores. This time I really questioned God's plan. Was I really doing His work by teaching sophomores to give injections and baths and medication? It only took me one year to know that this was where I was to be now, but inside I had a growing awareness that this was only preparation for a bigger plan. I honed my teaching skills and one day I was again dragged by a colleague to a church where the first parish nurses from Illinois were speaking. God spoke loud and clear to me that morning. This was what He was preparing me for. Only because I knew I was following God's lead, did I dare to prepare a curriculum for parish nurses, using the experience and knowledge I had been building.

My first class of parish nurses in 1990 was at Concordia University in Mequon, Wisconsin. I couldn't believe that God sent 19 women for me to teach. Should I have then written a five-year plan as to where my parish nurse curriculum would grow? Again, I didn't have the daring to foresee God's ten-year plan. I didn't give up my "day job," teaching sophomores for several years as the parish nurse program grew, drawing nurses from all over the country. After two years at Concordia, I transferred the program to Marquette. Four years ago, my dean wisely relieved my teaching assignment with sophomores and we created the Parish Nurse Preparation Institute. I became the Director.

Still I hadn't the courage to write a goal. Although my dean, like my earlier instructor, wishes I would. How could I have predicted that in ten years I would have educated over 1400 nurses to do God's work of healing in His congregations across the U.S., Mexico, and Canada? My plate seemed full with teaching parish nurses, but a Reverend Tom Paxton, as God's agent, introduced me to Ann Navera, the Director of Nurses at Sinai Samaritan Hospital. Together we joined our gifts and extended parish nursing into the first hospital parish nurse program in Wisconsin. My unwritten goal was to start the program, but seven years later I am still privileged to be part of this now bigger hospital system of Aurora Medical Services, serving forty some churches and a synagogue.

How could I have predicted that my life would be blessed to meet so many wonderful people that would never have been part of my life if I wasn't immersed in parish nursing education? Only by allowing the hand of God to write my five- and ten-year goals have I accomplished things my human mind would never have dreamed, never have written into that early nursing class.

So I feel safe today, in God's hands, without a written year goal for my future. With the past so rich in God's blessings, how could I fail to know there is a computer somewhere with the plans God has for the rest of my life? I see indicators of work for me with parish nursing in different parts of the world, as I meet parish nurses from Korea, Australia, Finland, and see opportunities to bring healing to the orphanage my daughter's church is building in Mexico. Like Samuel, I can only wait in the night and say, "Speak, Lord, for thy servant heareth".[14]

Janet Griffin's story provides another example of God's sometimes surprising work. As Janet looks back over her life she recognizes a series of transition points in her journey. At each transition, God's voice, hand, and guidance are the constants as she has dealt with the twists and turns in her life's journey.

AS AN ADULT, I faced a major career transition in the spring of 1986. I had been working as an instructor of practical nursing at a local community college. Because of declining enrollment, I was "pink slipped" and wondered where my professional life was headed. That summer while reading the want ads in the paper, I learned that a church in our area was looking for a "Minister of Health." Through that contact I became aware of the newly established parish nurse movement. By August, I was making regular trips to Des Moines, Iowa, to participate in Iowa Lutheran Hospital's Health Ministry Education Program, and began serving at St. Paul Lutheran Church in Davenport, Iowa.

As I began my new position, I had to consciously focus on "being with" people rather than "doing for," but a personal experience made a lasting impression. I was working at my desk in the church office one day when a call came from the hospital. A young woman from the congregation had been admitted because of an exacerbation of a chronic debilitating disease, and I was asked to visit her. When I entered her room, I sat next to her and held her hand. The doctor came in and explained a new treatment option; when he left, I clarified some details. The patient was very tired so my visit was short, but I before I left I offered a prayer.

As I returned to the church, I felt inadequate because I was concerned that I hadn't done anything for this young mother. Several weeks later, however, I received a call from her. She thanked me for being so helpful and said, "You prayed for me when I was too weak to pray for myself." The light bulb came on. I was now involved in a ministry of presence!

My four years at St. Paul were extremely rewarding, but

change was about to come my way again. My husband and I were facing the financial challenge of putting three children through college. I needed to give up my part-time job and seek a full-time position. So, in September 1990, I began working as Case Coordinator in the Senior Services Department at Trinity Medical Center in Moline, Illinois.

The job was not satisfying to me, but the hospital had recently started a Parish Nurse Program, so I enjoyed connecting with the director of that program, Harriet Olson. In October 1991, Harriet surprised me with the news that she needed a full-time Assistant Coordinator, and I was delighted to be appointed to that position. Then, just a year later, when Harriet decided that she didn't want full-time employment, I was named Director of Trinity's Parish Nurse Program. Wow! What an unexpected opportunity![15]

Sometimes we hear God's voice through the actions and words of others. The following nurses heard God calling them to parish nursing after attending a parish nurse conference. In 1992, Linda B. Martin (now Dr. Lynda W. Miller) was a doctoral student in the University of Victoria School of Nursing, British Columbia. Lynda traveled to the National Wellness Conference in Wisconsin, where she heard Ann Solari-Twadell, the director of the International Parish Nurse Resource Center in Illinois, describe a unique and innovative role of promoting healing and wholeness of individuals, families, and churches. The role described by Ann was of course that of a parish nurse. God used Ann to catch Lynda's attention; Lynda became one of Canada's parish nurse pioneers!

AT ONCE I KNEW I'd found a way to bring together all my experience as a professional nurse and as a member of the Christian faith community. I felt I could passionately devote myself as a whole person—spirit, soul and body—to this kind of nursing work for the rest of my life.[16] At my next meeting with my graduate program supervisor, I shared my excitement about parish nursing. My enthusiasm prompted her to suggest, "Then why don't you see if you can work it into your dissertation?"[17]

Kelly Preston also heard God calling her after attending a seminar on parish nursing.

HAVING WORKED on an oncology unit after graduating with my B.S.N., I sensed God calling me to utilize my nursing knowledge, my life experiences, and my faith in a different way. In fact, all throughout nursing school, I felt called to minister to the whole person, which is very difficult to do, unfortunately, in most clinical sites. I left my position at the hospital and began working at my church as an assistant to some of the pastors. The very week I started working at the church, I attended a seminar on parish nursing and health ministry. I don't believe this was a coincidence! From that moment on, I began praying and planning to share a proposal with our pastors about developing a health ministry in our church. God began to move and a few months later the pastors agreed to begin a health ministry, with me serving as the coordinator on a voluntary basis. It was a true answer to prayer! God continued to answer my prayers and I am now working as the Congregational Health Program coordinator for Baptist Health System in Alabama. We partner with faith communities of various denominations to develop health ministries and parish nurse programs. I truly feel this is what God has called me to do![18]

Other times the Lord's call comes in the midst of some activity that seems just as meaningful and the nurse's response is less than enthusiastic. Dianne Smith, a parish nurse consultant and health ministry educator, tells how she heard God calling her to parish nursing.

IN 1996, my eighty-two-year-old director of nursing at Florida Southern College knew that I taught ladies her age in my Sunday school class. She assigned me the topic of parish nursing for a paper that was due. I was angry because I had already chosen another topic and had completed my preliminary research. Because of my respect for her, I had an "attitude adjustment" and completed the paper on parish nursing. I was interested in the topic but the thought of nursing in a church environment scared me to death! I had *no* plan of doing this. God had other plans. He kept reintroducing me to the idea and eventually I could not think of another area of nursing that would be enjoyable.

This process took me about seven months. I have always felt that God does not call the trained, but trains the called. This is true in my case. I have not stopped in the last few years. More areas of parish nursing are evolving and I want to master them all. My practice has to be excellent because that is the only standard good enough for God and his people. I am currently speaking of parish nurse ministry versus parish nurse practice. This should not be an either/or proposition. The ministry is founded on a calling from God. It is as clear a spiritual calling as any heard by a pastor or evangelist. I always know when God is speaking to me because it is never the path or course I would have chosen. He always sends me to places I would not normally feel comfortable going to and puts me with people I would not have chosen to be with. When I listen to His voice, the situation turns out as He planned, and I am left thinking, *wow*, God is awesome![19]

Indeed, God is awesome. Gently and persistently He is calling His nurses. Some He speaks to directly; some He speaks to through dreams; some He speaks to through pain and discouragement; and others He speaks to through other nurses. Each hears His call and responds—not always knowing what this new uncharted journey will hold—but moving forward in faith nonetheless. Before going on to chapter 2, where we explore what God is calling nurses to, it is fitting to end this chapter with the words of a hymn entitled "Here I Am, Lord"—a summation of God's call to nurses and their response.

I, the Lord of sea and sky, I have heard my people cry.
All who dwell in dark and sin My hand will save.
I, who made the stars of night, I will make their darkness bright.
Who will bear my light to them? Whom shall I send?

I, the Lord of snow and rain, I have borne my people's pain.
I have wept for love of them. They turn away.
I will break their hearts of stone, Give them hearts for love
  alone.
I will speak my word to them. Whom shall I send?

I, the Lord of wind and flame, I will tend the poor and lame.
I will set a feast for them. My hand will save.
Finest bread I will provide, Till their hearts be satisfied.
I will give my life to them. Whom shall I send?

REFRAIN:

Here I am, Lord, Is it I, Lord? I have heard you calling in the
night. I will go, Lord, if you lead me. I will hold your people
in my heart.[20]

CHAPTER 2

Called to Serve

Ministry of Word and Action

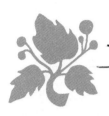 Parish nursing is a unique practice model in that nurses are called upon less for their "hands on" skills and much more for their "being with" skills. In chapter 1, Janet Griffin described her experience of praying with a young woman hospitalized for an exacerbation of a chronic debilitating disease as a "ministry of presence"—quite a departure from Janet's usual nursing practice.[1] The literature that describes parish nursing usually focuses on specific functions fulfilled by the nurse. There are a variety of descriptors with great overlap among writers. For instance, Granger Westberg used the term "minister of health" to describe the parish nurse and suggested four major functions: 1) health educator; 2) personal health counselor; 3) trainer of volunteers; and 4) organizer of support groups.[2] Since Westberg's original work three functions have been added: 1) referral agent and liaison with congregational and community resources; 2) integrator of faith and health; and 3) health advocate.[3] Joanne Sensenig, a parish nurse educator with the Mennonite Congregations, identifies similar functions.[4] In this chapter, we examine the seven combined functions.

We believe that all seven of these functions are part of two overlapping ministries: a ministry of action referring to "how the nurse does what is done" and speaking to the very essence of who the nurse is; and a ministry of word referring to all that the nurse says to the congregation in the way of education, advice, compassion, and advocacy.

Words paired with actions are a powerful combination—they go to the heart of genuine caring. When Janet Griffin prayed with the seriously ill young woman, Janet feared that she had not done enough. Shouldn't she have "done something to the patient"?—was her concern. Yet later the young woman thanked Janet for being so helpful and said, "You prayed for me when I was too weak to pray for myself." It was a very simple yet incredibly powerful intervention— Janet came to the hospital and she prayed. There are other seemingly simple interventions that carry the same powerful impact because of the message that is conveyed. Actions such as touching a congregant's arm to show compassion; shutting the door to an office to convey respect for the confidential nature of what is to be shared; making a telephone call on the anniversary of a loved one's death to console, remember, and honor; providing necessary health-related information to make informed decisions; praying for someone who is unable to form the words of supplication; making a "sick call" to someone who is in a hospital or nursing home or who is homebound; demonstrating respect for the decision making of another; being willing to accompany another on her journey even if that journey ends in death; a willingness to be a nonjudging listener; demonstrating humility in acknowledging the limitations of one's knowledge and a willingness to accompany another in seeking answers—these are all part of the ministries of action and word that when combined are so effective. Of course, these ministries are undergirded by professional knowledge that guides the nurse in making the appropriate decisions about how best to help the parishioner. Dianne Smith describes this best when she says, "My practice has to be excellent because that is the only standard good enough for God and His people."[5]

Let's return to the stories of parish nurses to discover how they describe their service in terms of the seven functions of health educator, personal health counselor, trainer of volunteers, organizer of

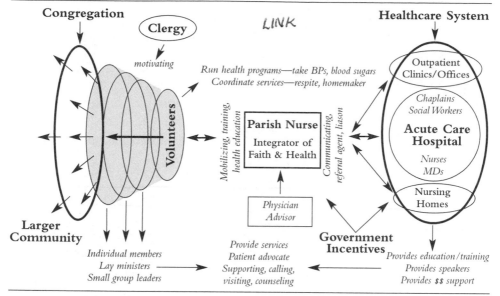

FIG. 2.1.Adapted from Koenig, H. (2001). Presented at the conference "Faith in the future: Religion, aging, and healthcare in the 21st century," Duke University, Durham, North Carolina.

support groups, referral agent and liaison with congregational and community resources, integrator of faith and health, and health advocate. The following figure illustrates the functions of the parish nurse as the nurse provides the vital link between the secular (health-care system) and the sacred (congregation).[6] As we discuss each of these functions we encourage you to refer to this figure.

Health Educator

Every article and book written about parish nursing highlights the function of health educator. Knowledge empowers people. Girded with adequate understanding, individuals are able to make good health-related decisions. These decisions include ways to preserve health through diet, exercise, and stress management; ways to manage health problems to minimize pain, discomfort, and disability; and ways to live with chronic health problems so that life continues to be a journey of joy and meaning.

All the nurses who shared their stories with us mentioned the importance of conducting blood pressure screenings. A rudimentary nursing procedure serves as an entrée not only into the lives of parishioners but also as an entree into the church community. Most nurses establish monthly or bimonthly blood pressure screenings, usually following one of the Sunday worship services. Many parishioners who would never voluntarily bare their souls to another find that through the blood pressure screening they are free to share what is most troubling to them. While the nurse collects valuable health information, she is able to educate at the same time.

Education is such an important function of the parish nurse that it is difficult to isolate specific "educational moments." Most nurses who shared their stories with us identified the many ways that they educate. For instance, there is the informal "one to one" contact where the nurse has the opportunity to teach while performing another task such as participating in health fairs or conducting screenings for blood pressure. Health education is also provided through educational seminars that are initiated by the parish nurse for the congregation. The parish nurse chooses the topics of these seminars after analyzing a needs assessment for the congregation.[7] Sometimes the nurse is the teacher; other times the nurse invites an expert from the community to share information with parishioners. Topics such as health-care proxies, funeral planning, bereavement, aging well, date rape, sexual abstinence, biblically based weight control programs, CPR instruction, wholistic heart health, male/female communication, stress and hope, are just a sampling of the types of presentations that are being given in churches where parish nursing is operational.[8] Furthermore, Buijs and Olson[9] believe that the parish nurse has an important role in providing education for families with young children.

In addition to the informal teaching and the formal seminars, parish nurses also fulfill the health educator function through the development and distribution of written materials, be they church bulletin inserts or resource centers stocked with both nurse-developed materials as well as those provided by professional organizations such as the American Heart Association. For example, Ellen Altenhofer assessed that the need was great for bereavement support and education. She developed bereavement follow-up packets for any congregational member(s) who had recently experienced a loss. This packet contains information regarding what grief feels like, how to cope with loss, how to answer the questions of a child about death, how to help a child deal with death, a list of community resources such as support groups, and literature on the grieving process. This packet of information is followed by actions such as sending sympathy cards to the family, making telephone calls at intervals of one month, six months, and one year; offering special support programs during the holidays; and presenting bereavement and loss inservices at the church.[10]

Deborah Baker extends the role of educator beyond the boundaries of her congregation.

> A UNIQUE ASPECT of the program is the partnership I have worked to create with Sonoma State University Department of Nursing. RN students with an interest in wholistic, faith-based practice have an opportunity to work with me during their community or senior-year clinical rotations. This benefits individuals and families from the congregation and community while providing a unique and maybe life-changing learning experience to nurses.

> A second prong to the development of the health ministry program at First Presbyterian Church has been the impetus to educate nurses, the religious community, and health systems within Sonoma County about the benefits of a parish nurse pro-

gram with a congregation. It was the first program to be developed in the county, and I have used it as a model for other congregations to follow in developing their own projects. Several times a year I am asked to speak about the role of the parish nurse to a variety of groups including ministerial associations, other congregations, groups of nurses, students in schools of nursing, and the local health systems. I feel as called to this aspect of education as I do to the actual role of parish nurse. I have a vision of the transforming power for the betterment of individuals and our community as a result of nursing practice that recognizes our interdependence, utilizes gifts of each individual, and looks creatively to build a healthy society. If every church had a parish nurse, and we all worked together to meet the unmet needs of the people, what a powerful force we could be![11]

Personal Health Counselor

Although the parish nurse function of personal health counselor overlaps significantly with the teaching role, counseling is almost always provided in a personal encounter between a parishioner and a parish nurse or a family and a parish nurse. Counseling certainly entails giving information, but the individual's or family's need is usually far deeper than factual exchange and involves dealing with lifestyle issues, as well as emotional and spiritual concerns that complicate health-care issues. In the following example Marianne Parker describes a need much deeper than the parishioner's request to participate in a blood pressure screening.

I REMEMBER one person who came to my hypertension screening. She had an elevated pressure. She was fearful to follow through with her physician because she was experiencing some of the same symptoms she had experienced immediately before her first stroke. Her family was encouraging her to see the doctor. She was afraid and in denial. We spoke about her symptoms. I provided her with information about the significance of these signs and encouraged her to seek follow-up care. We talked about her fears. We prayed together. When she left me she agreed to seek medical care. She left a more peaceful and affirmed woman.[12]

Marianne not only provided information, she provided counsel.

Trainer of Volunteers

We believe that of all the functions of the parish nurse, the training of volunteers may prove to be the most important service to the health-care system as we move forward in this century. Currently, the health-care system is struggling to provide adequate care and to contain costs. In 1966, when the Medicare system was first enacted, the total cost of the program per year was less than $5 billion. By 1980, it had increased to $38 billion, and by 1998, it had increased to over $200 billion per year. As the number of older adults in the population begins to increase dramatically after 2011 when 70 million baby boomers begin moving into the over sixty-five age range, projected growth and Medicare expenditures may swamp the health-care system's ability to provide. For example, the Department of Health and Human Services (DHHS) estimates that by 2007 the yearly Medicare budget will exceed $415 billion.[13] Bear in mind that this is *prior to* the rapid growth in the elderly population after 2011. Many would conclude that our medical system is broken. How then will this fragile system respond as the numbers of elderly increase from 35 million currently to 70 to 80 million in a few decades, along with a growing number of health problems, most of which are chronic conditions requiring a great deal of care?

The movement toward volunteerism or lay mobilization that is occurring across the country in many churches offers a hopeful response to this bleak picture. This movement is about the spirit of God working in His people to strengthen the work of God.[14] Parish nurses are in a wonderful position to mobilize and train church members of all ages. These volunteers are motivated by the highest goal to serve and honor their God by assisting one another and are the key resource within the church. They need to be utilized more fully. Furthermore, volunteering helps people to stay both mentally and physically healthy, according to a growing body of research in this area.[15]

Parker describes mobilizing volunteers as a three-step process: invite, ignite, and unite. This process goes beyond the creation and maintenance of a telephone-calling list of potential volunteers. *Inviting* involves helping the potential volunteer to see a clear vision and his or her unique role in that vision. The parish nurse must recognize that volunteer ministry experiences serve to highlight and uplift the personal journeys of each volunteer.[16] The parish nurse must honestly value each volunteer and believe that each one is a part of God's gift to the faith community.

Relationships are at the heart of lay ministry—the relationship between the volunteer and God, and the relationship between the volunteer and the parish nurse. Relationships require personal investment and regular tending. Although the invitation to lay ministry can be made through many avenues, including newsletters, church bulletins, pulpit invitations, and small group presentations, there is nothing that takes the place of a personal invitation with its power to communicate relationship and connection. An article in the *Catholic Review* quotes a study conducted by the Georgetown University Center for Applied Research in the Apostolate (CARA). This study profiled Catholics in the Washington, D.C., archdiocese and confirmed that "being invited" is by far the major reason why Catholics become active in their parishes. Furthermore, the study contends that if invitations to lay ministry from fellow parishioners and pastors were extended more, it would translate into at least a 10 percent increase in volunteers willing and even eager to contribute their skills and experience.[17]

As the parish nurse participates in recruiting volunteers, it is essential that the nurse listen for the message beyond the spoken words. Sometimes a response of "no" may require negotiation and clarification about exactly what is expected of someone who volunteers. It is essential that the minister fully supports the nurse's efforts to mobilize volunteers and, in particular, preaches *regularly* from the pulpit on the importance of volunteering as the role and responsibility of every Christian—"love thy neighbor," according to Jesus, was the only close second to the first commandment of "loving God." The Apostle John equated these commands entirely—"how can you love God, if you cannot love your fellow man right in front of you!"

Step two of the mobilization process is *igniting*, which focuses on training to build essential skills so that volunteers can succeed in their ministry settings. Training is needed so that those who volunteer their time know "how to listen," "how to support," "how to help the sick and disabled," "how to encourage independence," and "how to help the sick and disabled help others." All of these skills are considered part of nursing, but in the face of a nursing shortage, volunteers, under the guidance and supervision of the nurse, can provide many of these skills to their fellow parishioners. These services will help to maintain the chronically ill elderly in their homes, give them a sense of vision and purpose for their lives, and decrease the strain on the increasingly limited resources of the health-care system.

Using the word TRAIN, Parker describes the *igniting* phase in the following manner.

Teach the content in a manner and a time frame that values the experiences and other commitments of the volunteers.

Respect the time, talents, gifts, passions, questions, learning styles, and ideas of the volunteers.

Actively involve people during training. The nurse must model the ability to step out of a comfort zone and consider new behaviors and ways of interacting.

Ignite a renewed sense of God's call to ministry by focusing on purpose and passion.

Nurture the volunteers—they need to be cared about as they go about caring for others.[18]

Uniting is the third step of mobilizing volunteers. It is important for the nurse to unite the volunteers as a team. In addition to providing resources, encouragement, ownership, and affirmation of the volunteer's accomplishments, the parish nurse also can make use of buddy systems, team ministries, and mentoring opportunities that allow the volunteer to feel connected not only to the nurse but to the volunteer team.

In the fall of 1992, Ellen Altenhofer, parish nurse of Normandy Park Congregational Church, took a course entitled "Called to Care," which had been developed by the Office for Church Life and Leadership of the United Church of Christ. The "Called to Care" resource notebook includes a training program aimed at enhancing the skills of laypersons for ministries of caregiving. Terry Teigen, the pastor of Ellen's church, strongly advocated for the preparation of lay caregivers and worked with Ellen and others to develop a caregiving ministry. The "Called to Care" lay ministry was actually established before parish nursing was instituted. Laypersons were trained to provide support to members of the congregation during times of crisis, illness, or bereavement through the following activities: sending cards and notes; making hospital, home, or telephone visits; maintaining prayer chains; providing casseroles; providing transportation to doctor's appointments; and running errands. The lay volunteers were coordinated by Ellen and Joan Wieringa, another parish nurse. Additional volunteers were recruited from the congregation as needed, and along with the pastor, Ellen and Joan provided continuing education to increase the skills of the volunteers.[19]

Catherine Lomax reports,

I HAVE twenty-two "Friendly Visitors" from the church who visit with shut-ins, people living alone, and lonely people. They visit one to two times a month, send cards, and make telephone calls. They call me if they see any medical, social, or spiritual problems or questions that need answering. I meet with these wonderful people every three months to provide support.[20]

Most of the literature on parish nursing describes the value of volunteers in supporting the chronically ill elderly in their homes, but the value goes beyond this age group to encompass the needs of younger families as well. Buijs and Olson describe the use of volunteers to support young families with babysitting services as well as grocery shoppers, meal providers, and drivers. There exists the possibility of linking older parishioners who are isolated from their own families with children from other families within the church community—providing a surrogate grandparent-grandchild experience.[21]

Organizer of Support Groups

Support groups are a useful means to help individuals deal more effectively with a broad range of life stresses, from fighting an alcohol and/or substance abuse addiction to coping with the death of a young child. The power of the group to uphold its members, decrease their isolation, enhance their sense of connectedness, and enable them to gain new insights and differing perspectives gives support groups usually run by laypersons an important role in health. The role of the parish nurse includes organizing and facilitating support groups such as the Recovery from Loss group developed by Carole Kornelis. This group meets for nine weeks and deals with all aspects of loss, regardless of whether the loss occurred through death, divorce, unemployment, or the ending of a relationship.[22] Other times the parish nurse's role is to disseminate information to the congregation regarding already existing community-based support groups.

Referral Agent and Liaison

The role of the parish nurse is not to replace what is already being offered within a community but to assist parishioners to access existing appropriate resources to meet their particular needs. To fulfill this role the parish nurse must develop an in-depth knowledge of exactly what is available within the church community. For example, does the church provide volunteer services to assist with specific needs, such as home visitation, a food pantry, and/or short-term emergency funds for parishioners who are suffering financially? The nurse needs to know what is available within the surrounding community, such as flu shot clinics, free mammograms for breast cancer screening, home health care, and respite, homemaker, and transportation services. Additionally, the nurse must know how to access these resources, how these resources are paid for, whether they provide transportation, and what the waiting time is for appointments.

The nurse needs to communicate with hospital-based discharge planners, primary care physicians, specialists, clinics, and any other provider within the health-delivery system. Two other health-care specialists that the parish nurse must communicate with are chaplains and pastoral counselors. The role of the parish nurse may seem to compete or overlap with the role played by these religious leaders. However, there is much more room for complementation than competition. The needs for spiritual care can be so enormous that spiritual resources can be stretched to their limits. The primary domain of the chaplain and the pastoral counselor is the formal health-care setting (hospitals, nursing homes, outpatient clinics, etc.), whereas the primary domain of the parish nurse is the community (and more specifically, the religious community). There is tremendous need for the spiritual care delivered in the health-care setting to be continued in the patient's home, family, and religious environments. This will require close communication between chaplains and parish nurses, particularly around the time of hospital or nursing home admission, or hospital or clinic discharge. Each will find the other a tremendous, helpful resource as they strive to meet the patient's or family's spiritual needs on a continuous basis.

The nurse has a pivotal role in linking church members with these services and in helping them to navigate the turbulent waters of the health-care system. Marianne Parker notes the importance of parish nurse liaising not only with congregational and community resources but also with state and federal parish nurse contacts, which are essential to ensure that the nurse remains current about emerging trends, regulations, and resources that have a direct impact on the practice of parish nursing.[23]

Kelly Preston discusses a challenge confronted by many parish nurses because they are "referrers" and "linkers to care" rather than direct providers of care.

> WE HAD A YOUNG WOMAN from our church survive a terrible care wreck, which left her paralyzed from the neck down. She went through extensive surgeries and therapy, and is doing wonderfully today. However, during her days of therapy, her physician ordered a catheter to be placed so that she could go out of town for a few days with her family. The physician did not provide a means for this catheter to be inserted. I was torn because the family are good friends of mine, but at the same time, I knew that this type of invasive procedure was beyond the scope of parish nursing. I told the mother that I could not do it but would do my best to find someone who could. I contacted a home health nurse from our church who was also familiar with the family. The nurse felt perfectly comfortable doing this procedure. She also taught the mother how to take the catheter out when they returned from their trip. This was a challenge for me—recognizing my own boundaries and making sure the parishioner received the needed care.[24]

Dianne Smith discusses the need to have a structured process in place when making doctor referrals to a congregant.

> I ALWAYS GIVE three suggestions when I make doctor referrals. I give these in writing and tell the parishioner if I have had some contact with the physician or if I just know of his reputation as a skilled clinician. In this incident, a parishioner I was visiting had

been diagnosed with a bone spur, which turned out (too late!) to be cancer. His wife told me that "the doctor you recommended misdiagnosed his cancer as a bone spur." While she did not seem upset, the tone in her voice still worried me. I reminded her that I had suggested three different doctors and told her I had no experience with these physicians. I had suggested she ask around church and find someone who knew and had visited these doctors before she decided who to go to for medical care. The wife told me later that she had not meant to imply anything by her comment. I reassured her it was okay. I did feel better, however, knowing that I had followed protocol and had documented the referral appropriately. Just because you work in a church setting does not mean that you will not have others criticize you and even possibly threaten litigation.

Joyce McCasland, a parish nurse in Minnesota, reports that through her blood pressure screenings she frequently assesses a potentially serious problem that results in a referral.

A WOMAN was having dizzy spells that coincided with a very low pulse. I work full time in a cardiac care unit and was able to get her in to see a cardiologist. She ended up having a pacemaker implanted. She thought her dizzy spells were caused by stress and wasn't going to do anything about it. Another time I was doing blood pressure checks and one of the women had a very elevated BP. I encouraged her to see her doctor, which she did. The doctor increased her blood pressure medication and ordered a diuretic. She was so grateful—she said she would never have called the doctor if I hadn't suggested it.[25]

One of the initial activities of a new parish nurse is to become intimately acquainted with the health-care professionals and health-care centers used by church members. Telephone calls made to individual health-care practitioners allow parish nurses to introduce themselves, to provide a brief explanation of the role of the parish nurse in maintaining the health of the parishioner, and to request that the parish nurse be included in health-care planning so as to maintain a true continuity of care.

Integrator of Faith and Health

Every parish nurse who participated in this book emphasized two things: the importance of prayer at every juncture of her practice, and the need for constant awareness that parish nursing is God's work and He is in charge of every aspect of it. Many mentioned the necessity of praying for guidance when the call to parish nursing first becomes apparent; the need to pray as overtures are made to the congregation; the need to pray for acceptance by parishioners; the need to pray for wisdom as the parish nurse role is defined and communicated, and as boundaries are set; the need to pray as individual programs are developed, implemented, and evaluated; the need to pray for God's guidance in each nurse-parishioner encounter; and the need to pray to build the link between faith and health for the parish community. Clearly, the centrality of God, prayer, and faith are paramount in the practices of those who have been called to parish nursing. As Cheryl Hoviland says, "when you pray for someone, you begin to love them."[26]

Some of the most powerful stories shared by nurses were those that involved the integration of faith and health. Judy Shelly tells the following story:

> I HAD RECEIVED a phone call from one of our church members, "George," who had terminal cancer. He said he couldn't go on any longer and was ready to commit suicide. He was a hunter and had guns in the house. A widower who desperately missed his wife, George was lonely. He attended the monthly healing services at church but rarely attended the regular worship services.

I asked him to wait until I could come over. When I arrived, he was sitting in a recliner surrounded by five-foot high stacks of boxes containing formula for his gastric feedings. When I asked about his feeding, the amount seemed insufficient for adequate nutrition. He was barely using the supply of formula that he had available. He was in severe pain and getting poor relief from the medications prescribed. Although the visiting nurse came three times a week, he had not told her any of his concerns, which he now started to share.

After crushing an analgesic and injecting it into his gastrostomy, George began to talk about his fears and hopelessness. He was sure God was angry with him for not attending church and for the way he had treated others. After listening for about forty-five minutes, I asked if I could pray with him. His eyes lit up and he rose up from the chair. First he landed on his knees, and then lay prostrate on the floor. He began to pour out his heart to God, sobbing and visibly shaking. Frankly, I felt a bit frightened, not sure what was happening.

After about five minutes, George got up and sat peacefully back in his chair, and asked me to pray. He wept quietly, but seemed to glow with peace. After the prayer, as we were talking quietly, his brother arrived. I asked George if he could tell his brother about what was going on. I assured them both that George's despair seemed to have two very important physical aspects—poor pain control and hunger. We called the visiting nurse, who contacted George's physician to get both the pain medication and the feeding schedule adjusted.

George died peacefully in his sleep (of natural causes) about two weeks later.

Health Advocate

The last function to be discussed is that of health advocate—someone who supports and defends the position of the parishioner.

In today's fast paced and highly technological health-care system it is important to have an advocate who will speak and stand up for the parishioners health-care rights, values, and needs. It is also important that someone affirms and validates the desires of the parishioner's heart. Nadine Murphy in Alberta, Canada, performs the role of advocate by accompanying church members to doctor's appointments so that she is able to translate a diagnosis into terms that they can understand, or to lead them through the maze of the health-care system.[27]

Susan Dyess tells the story of Laura, a young woman who desperately needed an advocate, a person who could affirm the validity of her choice.

I DID NOT KNOW how to recognize Laura, but I had a preset notion based on her sister's brief description of her when she requested my visit. I had not yet spoken with Laura but was assured by her sister that my visit was desired.

I entered the facility and the door behind me locked. The unit appeared to be quiet. The unit also appeared to be bland, without color or character. The hallways were notably barren. The waiting room was also plain, no magazines, no books, nothing. There were only two walls and two panels of glass that allowed for viewing (or monitoring) from the nurse's station. There was a chair and a loveseat. An announcement broke the silence of the waiting room. Apparently a group session was about to begin and all were summoned to attend. I waited.

Laura appeared. She was a thin woman, with long blond hair and green eyes. She wore a black headband, street clothes, no makeup, and was remarkably well groomed. I would describe her as pretty. Her face was tear streaked, but she was not crying. She approached the waiting room with hesitation, but continued and there we met. We stayed in the waiting room so that we could have the most privacy.

Slowly, Laura began to disclose her situation to me. I listened. Laura was addicted to crack, and partied heavily. She was fighting a lifelong battle with poor self-esteem, and long-term battles with anorexia nervosa and bulimia. She had been abused by her father and her boyfriend. She was completely disgusted with her life and periodically thought of suicide. But Laura also expressed her desire and willingness to change. And then Laura shared the part I already knew (from what her sister had shared with me), that she was four weeks pregnant.

"Everyone is telling me to have an abortion," she said. "The doctor is, my father is, my boyfriend is . . . But they don't know. The doctor didn't even discuss it with me. He encouraged me to have an abortion and simply assumed I would. My boyfriend said he would have nothing to do with me; he doesn't want kids. My father said it would be best for everyone if I just had the abortion. I don't really believe in abortion. I have always wanted to have a child. But I am so messed up. I don't know if I could be a mother."

Laura began to sob. I held her and cried too.

Laura's tears came for a long time. Then she asked me a question as she gazed into my eyes: "Do you think it is selfish of me to want to keep this baby?"

The question pierced my soul. "No," I said.

From that moment, I knew Laura had made her decision. Laura chose life for her unborn baby.

Our shared time continued with a conversation exploring pregnancy, healthy living, and prenatal checkups. Laura had many questions. I attempted to provide information and direction for the questions. Her countenance changed as it began to sparkle.

My relationship with Laura was maintained by phone calls, letters, and brief interactions. After we met, Laura entered a six-month in-patient rehabilitation program. Months later, she gave birth to a healthy baby boy. Laura became a mother—she grew as a caring person. I did too.[28]

In summary, the parish nurse carries out a dual ministry of word and action to fulfill seven specific functions. These functions include health educator, personal health counselor, trainer of volunteers, organizer of support groups, referral agent and liaison with congregational and community resources, integrator of faith and health, and health advocate. The nurse's presence, compassion, knowledge, communication skills, and spiritual strength all combine to create a powerful ministry where the focus is more on "being with" and less on "doing for" the parishioner.

The next chapter examines the soaring mountain peaks when parish nurses say "this is why I became a nurse," and the valleys when parish nurses feel that the challenge of helping a parishioner is beyond their level of skill.

CHAPTER 3

The Journey of the Parish Nurse within the Church

Life is a journey of twists and turns, unexpected detours, unbelievable highs and unthinkable lows. So too is the journey of parish nursing. And like the journey of life, parish nursing holds incredible paradoxes—joy and sorrow, happiness and grief, excitement and frustration.[1] It is never boring. The parish nurse is granted the privilege of accompanying church members on parts of their lives' journeys. Sometimes the nurse is invited into the private and intimate world of parishioners. In response to this invitation, the parish nurse frequently facilitates transformative healing, both in the individual as well as in the family. At other times, the invitation brings the nurse in direct confrontation with a magnitude of pain and unmet needs that is not only overwhelming but leads the nurse to question her ability to make a difference. The parish nurse is drawn to offer whatever is possible to ease suffering, provide reassurance, facilitate peace, bring about reconciliation, increase coping, and enhance spiritual well-being—certainly not easy tasks. However, when we asked nurses to describe the highs and lows, the joys and challenges of their journeys, the most common theme was, "Now I know why God called me to become a nurse!"

Challenges of the Journey

Overwhelmingly, nurses responded to the question regarding their challenges in health ministry with seven themes: 1) the nurse encounters general resistance to the concept that healing is part of the church's ministry and specific resistance to the idea that the parish nurse can be an integral resource in the church's reclamation of that ministry; 2) the needs of church members exceed the boundaries of the parish nurse role and sometimes the abilities of the nurse; 3) the assessed needs of church members exceed the time available for ministry; 4) the nurse's vision for ministry differs from the congregation's expectations, resulting in "expectation conflict"; 5) the community at large lacks understanding about the body-mind-spirit focus of the parish nurse and expects the nurse to function as a community health nurse and the church as another community agency; 6) the parish nurse often confronts territorial jealousy from other church staff members; and 7) the parish nurse often experiences professional isolation unless the nurse is part of a network of parish nurses.

Resistance to Parish Nursing

Dianne Smith provides advice to nurses confronting the challenge of "selling parish nursing" to a congregation.

MY BELIEF is that the first step in convincing a church that parish nursing is a wonderful addition to the ministry team is to pray. The second, third, and fourth steps include education, education, and more education! Establishing the structure of a health ministry team, cabinet, or committee is another essential step before parish nursing can begin to flourish. This team/cabinet provides the nurse's base of support and a body of people both interested in health ministry and willing to help enlist the workers that will be needed to meet the needs of the congregation effectively. The nurse then provides an umbrella of "health expertise" over the ministry for the congregation.

Most pastors have a basic knowledge of the scriptural commands regarding health, healing, and wholeness, but they are frequently so stretched that they are not able to devote their energies to this ministry. I found that the easiest way to sell pastors on the idea of parish nursing is to approach them from the perspective that parish nursing is an effective way to decrease the demands placed upon them. For instance, preventive health measures such as blood pressure screenings offered by the nurse have a direct impact on the health of church members. A parishioner who becomes aware of high blood pressure and gets treatment is less likely to end up in the hospital with a stroke. Congregants who are convinced to wear their seat belts and sit at least eleven inches (the length of a sheet of copy paper) away from the airbag will probably not be as severely injured in a possible automotive accident as people who do not wear seat belts or who sit too close to the airbag. In addition, the parish nurse can visit many of the parishioners who become hospitalized or are homebound. Having a nurse on staff offers another bonus for the pastor because the nurse is able to counsel some of the people the pastor is not capable of or comfortable counseling.

Another challenge that I have confronted is that the very person who is the most resistant to the parish nurse ministry can become the most ardent supporter. For example, a gentleman in my church adamantly opposed the idea of a health ministry. He didn't believe it was the church's role to meddle in the health of congregants. Amazingly, within two months after I had proposed the role of parish nurse, his wife became seriously ill. I visited and offered help in weaving through the maze of their HMO. It became obvious to me that the wife needed a transfer to a medical teaching center for a more extensive work-up. Initially the HMO refused this request. I sat in on a meeting that included the husband and representatives of the HMO. I offered my support to the family and advocated for the transfer of his wife to another facility. Within twenty-four hours the transfer order had been written. Sadly, she died before a definitive diagnosis could be made. However, from that point on this gentleman sang the praises of parish nursing. The man who had presented the biggest challenge that I had faced in establishing the parish nurse ministry became a walking advertisement. Because he had been so vocal in his opposition to parish nursing, his changed heart made others take note and want to know more about the ministry.[2]

Kristine Holmes describes a similar story of challenge when parish nursing was first introduced to her congregation. She met resistance from quite a few influential individuals and families in her church who saw no need for parish nursing. What Kristine calls "GMCs"—God Made Coincidences—helped her to overcome this challenge of resistance.[3]

> LET ME DESCRIBE two of the stories. There was one older, retired couple who had been members of the church for many years. They had the attitude, "We never had a parish nurse before, we never needed one before, why do we need a parish nurse now—especially since there is money involved." (This concern about cost was totally unfounded since I was unpaid for three years and when I became salaried in 2000 the monies came from two grants.) Then the gentleman developed chest pain and ended up at the local community hospital. I went to visit this couple in the holding area while he was waiting to be transferred to a large medical center. I was timid and fearful because I knew their feelings about the program and me. When I walked in his wife threw her arms around me, began to cry, and then told me how grateful she was that I was there. I was able to explain the procedures that he would undergo, visit with him and the family, and after his successful angioplasty visited regularly to provide health-teaching materials on lifestyle changes. Since then he has had extensive surgery and has requested that I come to visit and be there after the surgery to provide support to him and his wife. Recently I overheard this couple defend parish nursing and the health ministry adamantly to a new couple

who had just joined our church and had questions about the ministry.

The second story is about another older couple who had been quietly opposing the parish nurse ministry. The wife came to see me one day to talk about her concern over changes she saw in her own behavior. She had once been active in the church and involved in lots of services. She no longer felt this enthusiasm and energy and was chronically sad. I assessed that she was probably depressed. I referred her to a geriatric psychiatric nurse clinical specialist for evaluation. Six weeks later she came back to see me, put her arm around me, and whispered, "Thank you. I am getting better. I feel like me again." This couple became part of my support and the lady became an active member of the health ministry team.[4]

Needs Exceed Boundaries and Abilities

Anna Friedberg describes a different type of challenge—one where the needs swamp resources and abilities. She feels deeply for the needs of the youth in her church.

MANY OF THE YOUNGSTERS are from homes of pain and discord; abuse is part of their lives. Frequently these homes are the focus of child protective services. The children desperately need love; their families desperately need help. The church provides a safe haven, a place where love is freely given; yet it seems that it is too little. Our efforts to reach families are generally unsuccessful. We continue to love and care for the children. Many times when they are at church they don't want to go home.

Anna defines this as a dual challenge, not only to reach out to the children and their families but also to encourage those who volunteer so they do not lose heart for this ministry.[5]

Karen Thornton also describes a situation where the needs of a parishioner were greater than Karen's perceived abilities.

I VISITED an elderly woman and her caregiver daughter in their home. The tension between the two was palpable. They had a long history of unreconciled differences, and the current burden of caring for her mother left the daughter feeling very angry. I consulted with a medical social worker at the home care agency providing nursing care for the mother. I sat, listened, and tried to be supportive and understanding. I also arranged some respite care so the daughter was able to get out of the house. There was nothing I could do to fix this situation. Shortly after I became involved, the mother died with so many emotional and spiritual wounds unhealed.[6]

Ellen Kirker tells of two crises that occurred within minutes of each other during a church service.

ON PALM SUNDAY I was at Mass sitting at the back of church—it was blood pressure Sunday. It was a long service, very hot, and the smell of the incense was strong. Many parishioners were standing, including a lot of elderly people. In a row across from me a woman passed out and hit the floor. I attended her and made sure medics were called. Within five minutes another woman did the same thing on the other side of the church! To say it was a challenging situation is an understatement. I tried to respond to both women, coordinate the responding medic units, and then do the follow-up. Both women lived alone with no family in the area. I felt stretched to make sure they were both okay; I visited them in the hospital and coordinated their after-care.[7]

Other parish nurses shared this same challenge as well as their responses to it. For many, either the fear of or the actual experience of multiple crises occurring simultaneously within a church service was the impetus to develop an emergency response team charged with specific duties and responsibilities. Margie Maddox contacted the

American Red Cross and arranged for them to provide a program for church ushers, "What to Do Until Help Arrives." This program was developed for nonmedical people waiting for emergency personnel to arrive after dialing 911.[8]

Linda Whitesell describes feeling inadequate when helping church members make informed decisions regarding their healthcare insurance.

> I VISITED an elderly homebound couple who had asked me to come see them. They were in distress because they were being forced to change their insurance plan from a less expensive HMO to a regular and much more expensive Medicare supplement. They asked my advice about various plans and where they could get additional information. I told them what I knew, but I felt frustrated that their options were so limited. The bottom line was that the Medicare supplement would cost them significantly more than they were currently paying and more than they could comfortably afford. Although they were appreciative that they had someone to talk to about this situation, I felt that I didn't help them very much.[9]

Needs Exceed Available Time

The third theme of challenge emerging from the nurses' stories is the limitation of time. The majority of parish nurses hold unpaid positions at their churches and at the same time are employed full time elsewhere. They juggle multiple demands. As they become increasingly aware of the needs that exist in their church community, they must confront their own time and resource limitations in responding to these needs. One of the nurses who shared her story encourages parish nurses to start small and to accept that it may not be possible to meet all of the assessed needs.

> WE STARTED with a great deal of enthusiasm and perhaps too much vision. In the first year we began taking blood pressures

monthly, sponsored a small health fair, taught a CPR course, assisted with a monthly healing service, developed a resource file with information about common medical problems, stocked the church library with health-related books, took responsibility for stocking the church first-aid kits, taught Sunday school teachers about universal precautions, created bulletin boards that changed with the seasons, and wrote monthly articles for the church newsletter!

By the second year, our number of nurses began to dwindle. Most were just too busy with their full-time jobs and families to invest in the parish nurse ministry. Three of us continued with the blood pressure screenings and a less ambitious level of programming. Most of the coordination and follow-through fell on me, although the other two nurses were always willing to do specific tasks when asked. However, even the blood pressure screenings created a growing awareness of needs—for counseling and support groups (especially in regard to abuse issues and grief), for teaching and encouragement (e.g., diet and weight control, healthy lifestyle), and for follow-up after hospitalization. The growing trust that developed with the personal contact involved with the blood pressure screenings also created a sense of openness in sharing concerns and crises.

We are now in our sixth year. Ideally, we could use a parish nurse at least twenty hours a week. I can't commit to that, so many of the assessed needs will not be met; however, I have sensed the Lord's direction to respond selectively in numerous situations.

This is a situation that confronts many parish nurses; they try to do everything by themselves. Naturally this leads to burnout. When the needs are great and the workers are few, the nurse is called upon—not to do more by herself, but to mobilize volunteers from within the congregation. This calling forth of volunteers must not be just the parish nurse's response to overwhelming needs; more importantly, it must also be the pastor's response from the pulpit. During the service, the pastor must directly encourage congregants to volunteer their time to help out in the health ministry. Perhaps even a show of hands during the service of who is willing to volunteer would get an immediate commitment! Without such support, parish nurses will invariably become overwhelmed with the magnitude of need in the congregation.

Expectation Conflict

The fourth theme of challenge emerging from the nurses' stories deals with "expectation conflict." Usually the parish nurse responds to a call from God that includes a very specific vision for the health ministry. Sometimes the nurse's vision is very different from what the congregation expects. All of the nurses who shared their stories participated in some type of formal parish nurse preparation that informed them regarding the role, definition, and functions of parish nursing. The nurses are clear that the scope of practice does not include the direct provision of physical care, but when needs for direct care arise in the congregation and are unmet, nurses feel an emotional tug to go beyond the defined boundaries of parish nursing. At times church members put pressure on the nurse to perform skills that more appropriately fall into a home health agency's domain.

Another nurse describes a different type of "expectation conflict." She was functioning as an unpaid parish nurse when she had a vision that was different from that held by the leadership of her church. This experience also highlights the importance of responding obediently to God's call.

I TRULY HAD A PASSION for the growth of a healing ministry at our church that would unleash the use of an individual's gifts for God's service. My perspective was strongly in the healing realm, which made sense, since that was my gift and passion. The leadership of my church had a vision and priority for small group ministry. When I tried to join myself to the vision held by the leadership and at the same time tried to hold onto the other passions to which I felt called, I quickly experienced the effects of spreading myself too thin. Clearly, God was calling me to ministry outside of the church family that I held so dear. I didn't want to hear that from Him. I wanted to stay where I was comfortable, where relationships had been fulfilling. Sadly, I learned that when I don't listen to God's call, I open myself to many negative human emotions. I also learned that as a parish nurse it is essential that I be aware of my own needs for healing and growth.[10]

Community Agencies Expect a Community Health Nurse

One of the roles of the parish nurse involves reaching out to the community at large and forging relationships with community-based providers. This reaching out provides the necessary link between the church community and outside health-based resources. Kristine Holmes describes the misunderstandings that arose when she began to reach out to the community.

> I SYSTEMATICALLY made contact with as many community health agencies as I could. I wanted them to know that I was working out of my church and that I might be contacting them periodically for information or to refer a church member for services. Almost immediately the local county health and human service agencies, as well as for-profit companies, were eager to establish relationships with the church. Many "holistic" businesses wanted to advertise or sell their products or services. I fielded many calls on topics that included magnet therapy, homeopathic medicine, and chiropractic services. The local health agencies wanted to provide information on the types of services and educational programs that they offered. The area hospitals were interested in promoting their wellness centers and physician referral services. Retirement communities and assisted living facilities were eager to give tours and complimentary meals.

Much of this information is good. However, it can be overwhelming and must be evaluated carefully. Agencies, businesses, and vendors view parish nurse/health ministry programs as a way to launch or promote their particular services or products. These services may indeed be beneficial, but it is important for the parish nurse to sort the wheat from the chaff. A congregation depends on the parish nurse to give honest, reliable information.

As I talked about the parish nurse role with health-care providers in the community, it was very clear that they just didn't get it. First of all, they struggled to see a difference between my role and that of a public health nurse. Secondly, they failed to see the wholistic nature of what I do—the integration of body, mind, and spirit. My church has helped me deal with this situation. There is a written policy that makes it clear that commercial businesses are not allowed to sell their products on church property. Likewise, I have invited guest speakers to lecture on specific topics, but with instructions that they are not to sell or promote their services or products. The education of community-based providers has been an ongoing challenge—one that I have committed myself to confronting with lots of education.

Territorial Jealousy

The role of the parish nurse is still unknown to many within the church. Although the skills of the nurse only add to the effectiveness of a church's health ministry, there are some who feel emotionally threatened by the nurse and what she is able to do. Giving up or sharing responsibilities with the nurse is sometimes greatly resisted. Ruth Stoll encountered this territorial jealousy when she worked as a parish nurse at St. Stephen's Episcopal Cathedral in Harrisburg, Pennsylvania, from 1996–2000.

WHEN I STARTED at St. Stephen's one of the deacons was responsible for all of the home visitation. I saw this as an important part of my role as well. How else would I be able to assess the wholistic needs of homebound church members? Initially the deacon was very slow to relinquish any of the visits to me. As I strategized about ways to approach him, I thought that I might be able to decrease his sense of threat if I asked to accompany him on his visits. I suggested that this would be a great way for me to get to know the congregation and also to learn from him. This softened him somewhat. His next tactic in guarding his territory was to "give" me the visits that he didn't want to do. This was a tough issue. It took over a year to resolve this problem fully. I hear other nurses face similar challenges. Sometimes it is a deacon who feels threatened; other times it is the pastor. Regardless, it can be a daunting challenge to deal effectively with the insecurity and fear felt by the individual putting up the roadblock and to move ahead with the parish nurse role.[11]

Professional Isolation

The sixth challenge focuses on the issue of professional isolation. In some areas of the country there are so few parish nurses that an individual nurse can feel very alone and on her own. Debbie Hyder from Kingston, Tennessee, experiences this challenge. Debbie's church is in a rural area in East Tennessee, in what Debbie calls "mountain culture"—by and large a culture of friendly, deeply religious people, who consider each other family, and who interact with loose formalities. Most of the residents live on farms at a distance from one another but they are linked by a strong sense of community, nestled firmly within the "Bible Belt" of the nation. Debbie's base of operations is a small office tucked away in the library of her church, Bethel Presbyterian USA, in Kingston.

ALTHOUGH I reach out to the surrounding community, I basically serve my church members. They do not all live in Kingston—they are spread far and wide across a three-county area. Although there are parish nurses forty-five miles away in Knoxville, Tennessee, I am the only parish nurse in the immediate area. I read everything I can get my hands on about parish nursing and I try to interpret this information to apply it to my church community. I use church surveys to assess needs of my church members. But, sometimes I feel like I am wandering in the dark—I know what the books say about parish nursing—but I don't always know if I am doing the right thing or enough of the right thing. I wonder if other parish nurses are doing what I am doing. I am hoping that my church's recent decision to support me by paying my expenses when I attend parish nurse conferences will help me to develop a network of parish nurses that I can draw on for support.[12]

This sense of professional isolation is also a risk when the nurse is the coordinator of a network of parish nurses. In this role a great deal of time is spent in an office alone. Perhaps this is the burden of leadership, but it remains a challenge. Again, let's hear from Marianne Parker.

MY MOST CHALLENGING experience as a paid hospital-based parish nursing program coordinator is working alone. I spend many hours in an office with limited contact with volunteers or the public. I have an outgoing nature and this aloneness is at times overwhelming. Although other staff people at the hospital participate in the wellness program, I am the only person working toward faith-based health promotion goals. I am in contact with parish nurses throughout our network; I consult with them and minister to them, but there is nobody at my level to do the same for me.

Joys of the Journey

By far, nurses shared more stories of joy than challenge. The stories encompassed eight themes: 1) providing necessary support and information to cope with difficult life circumstances; 2) facilitating family healing; 3) facilitating reconciliation with God and the church; 4) accompanying another along a journey of pain and uncertainty; 5) assisting another toward a peaceful death; 6) facilitating an unexpected healing; 7) making the right connections between people; and 8) bringing together a community of healing. Throughout these stories is woven the importance of spiritual care and specifically the importance of prayer.

Providing Necessary Support and Information to Cope

Linda Whitesell shares her successful implementation of a retreat for the women in her congregation.

> I SUGGESTED that the retreat focus on our own aging and the demands of caregiving for elderly parents. I recommended speakers who were nurses I knew and offered to speak myself. It was right up my alley since I am a geriatric nurse practitioner. The retreat was well attended and received. It filled a real knowledge void. So many women not only struggle with their own aging issues but also with the changing needs of elderly parents. Most of the women were unaware of normal aging. Furthermore, they really didn't know what was involved in being a caregiver, nor did they know where to turn for assistance. They were appreciative of the concrete information that we provided.

Facilitating a Family Healing

Carole Kornelis shares a situation involving a child-parent issue.

> A TWELVE-YEAR-OLD CHILD who attended our church was exhibiting destructive behaviors. His mother had taken him to work with her the day before to provide some direct oversight of his behavior, but he had spent much time alone in the car. He was bored and attempted to take things apart. His "mechanical efforts" resulted in the breakage of the radio and a few other mi-

nor things. The mother did not notice these broken items as she was driving home from work that day. However, the next day she again took her son to work with her and noticed the damage. She became very upset not only over the car problems but also over the realization that she would have to share this situation with her husband, her son's stepdad. She thought that her husband would become very angry with the boy—he didn't have a positive relationship with the young man. Without thinking, the mother stopped the car, ordered her son out of the car, and told him to walk the rest of the way to her workplace. She continued her drive to work. Arriving at work and realizing the foolishness of what she had done, she retraced her route trying to find her son. When she couldn't find him she called 911 and reported what had happened. She felt sheer panic at the thought of what could happen to her son, whom she described as very impulsive and irresponsible. Meanwhile, after the boy had gotten out of his mother's car, he had stopped at a farmhouse and had talked to the people living there. They were mystified as to why this child was out in this rural setting by himself. As they gathered information from the boy he told them what church he went to; a phone call was made to the church—where I got involved. I arranged to have him picked up—then called the mother and the police. The family was linked to social services and a family therapist. I was able to get the mother into a parenting class and her son into a social skills class. I had such a sense of satisfaction that when this boy was in need he thought of calling his church.[13]

Facilitating Reconciliation with God and the Church

Judy Shelly shares Susan's story—a story of reconciliation and healing.

SUSAN APPEARED on my doorstep after receiving radiation therapy for a rapidly growing thyroid cancer. Despite the cancer,

Susan expressed joy and great appreciation for life. But it wasn't always so. As a young woman Susan had been active in her church with a deep relationship with God. This changed when she had a serious disagreement with her pastor. Susan's anger was directed not only at the pastor but she also became angry and bitter towards God. She severed her relationship with the church.

Several years after Susan left the church her husband returned. He requested prayers for Susan that God might heal her of her bitterness and return to church with him. Once in a while she would come to a service, but she kept God and everyone else at a distance. Then Susan began to experience tragedy in her life. First, a son died in an automobile accident. Shortly thereafter Susan's brother died of cancer. Within a few months of her brother's death, Susan faced the same diagnosis.

Throughout all these crises, the church ministered to Susan—we sent her notes and flowers; I visited her regularly; and we prayed for her. She came back to God and to the church community. Even though Susan was dying, she had achieved a state of wholeness—and I had been instrumental in that, as was my church.[14]

Stories of reconciliation with God and the church seem to hold special significance for the parish nurse. Perhaps this is because most nurses are denied these opportunities in the current health-care system, which is oriented to symptom reduction rather than wholeness. This deficit in the health-care system fuels dissatisfaction among nurses and leaves patients and families with an overwhelming sense that their care has been inadequate.

Ellen Kirker was visiting a congregant in the hospital following surgery. Ellen believes that God used her visits to communicate an invitation to come back to church.

ONE OF OUR church members had serious surgery that she came through with flying colors. She had pulled away from the church years before. I visited her several times during her hospitalization. We prayed together every visit and the prayer seemed to produce joy on her face and relaxation in her body. She believed that through my visits God was giving her a second chance. She asked to speak to our pastor and to get reacquainted with the church. It was such a privilege to be used by God to assist this woman back to a relationship with God as well as her church community.

Accompanying Another along a Journey of Pain and Uncertainty

Many times congregational nurses are present as a church member journeys through a time of intense pain and sorrow. This is a privileged and sacred opportunity. The nurse is called to "be with" rather than to "do for" the individual. There are usually no specific skills or tricks of the nursing trade to make the situation better, to fix it, or to make the pain go away. The nurse is called on to be a witness, to be a fellow sojourner, and to support with presence, prayer, and patience. The nurse is called upon to draw on her own reserves of courage as she looks in the face of incredible loss, death, anguish, and grief. Words are futile; only presence is fruitful.

Catherine Licks describes a situation where she was called to accompany a young couple as they prepared for the birth of their child.

MY FIRST HOSPITAL VISIT as a parish nurse will always stay fresh in my memory. I felt that this was a confirmation from the Lord of my ministry. On a Friday afternoon, the church secretary called and said that a parishioner was in the hospital, in labor, but that the baby was dead. She said that the pastor was out of town and asked if I could visit.

Prayer was my companion all the way to the hospital. I asked the Lord to make me His instrument and to use me to serve and comfort this family. Upon arrival at the hospital I met the young woman, her husband, and several other family members. Talking to the husband, I discovered that the baby had stopped moving on Tuesday, and his wife had had an ultrasound on Wednesday. The doctor had hoped that labor would start spontaneously, but when it didn't he admitted her to the hospital and induced labor on Thursday. It was now late Friday afternoon and she was still in labor.

I was able to speak to Laura and Dan and reinforced the importance of seeing their baby after he was delivered. Also, during Laura's contractions I offered support and encouragement. I offered to pray with them, and uttered a simple prayer, "Lord, we don't know why this is happening. Our hearts are just breaking, but we know that you are in control and that you promise to be with us always. We pray that you will deliver this baby quickly and support Laura and Dan with your love and comfort." Soon after, I left the hospital. The next morning I received a call from Dan. He said, "Thank you so much for coming—what a miraculous answer to prayer; about two minutes after you left Laura delivered the baby!"

Over the next weeks, I continued to minister to Laura and Dan through visits, prayer, and the sharing of resources. This is a sad story in that a family suffered the loss of a baby, but it brought joy in that I saw how the Lord could use me as a nurse, a woman, and a Christian to minister to His people in times of greatest need.

As I reflect on this story I am reminded of something that Mother Teresa once said when a rich nobleman asked her whether or not she became discouraged because she saw so few successes in her ministry. Mother Teresa answered, "No, I do not become discouraged. You see, God has not called me to a ministry of success. He has called me to a ministry of mercy." In parish nursing, I am not called to preach or teach to hundreds of persons simultaneously. I hold one hand and hug one person at a time. I encourage one family awaiting the death of a parent or I sit with one family awaiting the return of a loved one from surgery. Parish nursing will never be a ministry of huge numbers, but a ministry of mercy, one person at a time.[15]

Catherine Lomax relates a similar story of journeying with a couple who had a difficult pregnancy.

ONE OF OUR church members, a thirty-six-year-old woman, had a very hard pregnancy. She had fibroids growing inside her uterus as well as outside the uterus in the abdomen. These fibroids produced a great deal of bleeding throughout the pregnancy, resulting in hospitalizations and bed rest. The woman was told that for her own health and well-being this had to be her only pregnancy. She ended up having a C-section and delivered a perfect and beautiful little girl, Lauren Nicole, who is a delight and a treasure. I had the privilege of walking through the pregnancy, delivery, and Lauren's baptism with this couple. I was able to support them with my presence, my prayers, my knowledge of obstetrics (I was a midwife in England for four years), and my ability to mobilize help for them. This was a very special time for me.[16]

Assisting Another toward a Peaceful Death

Catherine Lomax tells another story about visiting a dying parishioner in her home.

A FORTY-SEVEN-YEAR-OLD LADY in my church had bladder and kidney cancer with metastasis to her bones. The cancer was very aggressive and was spreading faster than she could get treatment. She was at home and had visiting nurses seeing her for hospice care. When I visited her she had tubes everywhere—in her bladder, kidneys, and abdomen. She had intravenous lines running for medication administration. She had sores in her mouth and had lost most of her hair. Only her strong faith and belief that she would get better kept her going. The day I visited her I found her crying—all of her tubes were leaking, and she was in pain and feeling absolutely miserable. I could not find a word of comfort for her in the ravages of this cancer, so I sat down next to her on the wet couch, put my arms around her, and we both cried. Out of this miserable situation she started to say the Lord's Prayer and together we got through it. She shared with me that she had three daughters, each of whom was pregnant. She wanted very much to be able to see these grandchildren born. One of her daughters delivered early and immediately faxed a picture of the baby to her mother. The mother was thrilled beyond words to have been able to see her first granddaughter. Two days later she quietly passed away at home in her own bed with all of her family with her.[17]

Karen Thornton shares another story of assisting someone toward a peaceful death.

MY MOST TOUCHING experience came soon after I became a parish nurse. Our pastor was out of town and I visited a dying church member in the hospital. I had known this gentleman and his family for over fifteen years—our children had grown up together. I was able to talk to him about what he wanted at the end of life. He asked for an explanation about what a "do not resuscitate" order meant. Because I had a long-term relationship with this family, they trusted me and felt at ease with my presence. I was able to give him and his family unlimited time and support. It was such a special privilege to be with them at this very important and yet sorrowful time. I knew that my interventions, my presence, my words, and my prayers were a real help to the gentleman as he accepted his own death as well as to the family as they let go of their loved one into the arms of God.[18]

Facilitating an Unexpected Healing

Terrill Stumpf relates a story from his days as a parish nurse in San Francisco.

I WAS A PARISH NURSE at Old First Presbyterian Church and working one day a week at the Seniors Activity Center—I had open office hours every Monday. One of the former members (an eighty-year-old woman) of the center had recently moved out of state and she was back in San Francisco on vacation. She stopped by the center to see me. We were having a friendly chat and catching up when she told me that she had been depressed and was taking an antidepressant medication about which she had questions. So I looked up the medication in a drug reference book—I checked indications, side effects, etc., and I shared this information in terms she could understand. As I was reviewing precautions for taking this medication, I pulled my glasses down on my nose (this was before I admitted to needing bifocals) and said teasingly that she shouldn't take this medication if she was pregnant. She looked at me, her face clouded over, and her eyes began to tear. I asked a probing question about the meaning of her tears and she began to relay a story of pain, guilt, and betrayal.

When she was twenty years old she had a relationship with a man who forced her to engage in sex. This happened again with a different young man when she was twenty-five. Both of these encounters resulted in pregnancy. Both times she was forced to move away from her hometown because of the shame of being pregnant and unmarried. She carried two daughters to term and then gave both of them up for adoption. For the last sixty years she had carried enormous guilt not only for becoming pregnant outside of marriage but also for giving up her children. She told me that because of the stigma, her sense of sinfulness, and the intense guilt that she felt she had never shared her story with anyone, including her pastors. When she moved out of San Francisco, she set about to locate her two daughters. She discovered that they were both living in the state where she had relocated. She contacted them separately, and she received very warm receptions from both daughters. As she was telling me this part of the story, her face glowed with a sense of peace. I was struck with the fact that even though she had carried this guilt for all these years, in reconnecting with her daughters she had achieved a degree of peace that could carry her through the remaining years of her life. I told her that I believed that God had really gifted her with His grace and that this grace must provide some sense of relief for her guilt. With that we both started crying.

Often I think that parish nurses get so caught up in our tasks that we miss opportunities to open windows to spiritual healing. If I had not used a bit of humor regarding her need to be cautious about pregnancy, would I have been able to open the window that allowed her to express her guilt and sorrow? After all these years she still carried guilt about giving up her daughters, about getting pregnant when she wasn't married, about feeling angry and betrayed at the hands of two men who had taken advantage of her. As a nurse one part of me felt that I should explore other parts of her story—like how she had handled this situation with her own parents—and had these situations affected her decision to get married or not—but I decided to just let her lead the conversation and share what she wanted to share. We ended up praying before she left and we said that we would see each other in church that Sunday. Sadly, I didn't see her Sunday and we never saw each other again. But when she left she had a glow on her face and I said, "Let the healing begin." As I reflected on this encounter, I felt that we had shared sacred space; I felt both humbled and at the same time very honored that she had shared this information with me.[19]

Kelly Preston discusses an unexpected healing that resulted from a stress management seminar sponsored by the Baptist Health System in Alabama.

ONE OF THE first things that we did at our church was to hold a stress management seminar. We had done a needs assessment and stress management was identified as the top need and priority. As we planned for this seminar we thought maybe thirty people would attend. To our great surprise nearly two hundred people came! We had a counselor from our church speak, as well as a couple of singers who sang songs that dealt with turning our lives and our cares over to the Lord. The immediate response from participants was that the seminar had been a real blessing. However the biggest blessing came after the seminar. I received an e-mail from a lady who had come from out of town to attend the seminar, stating that she wanted to hear one of the singers. But after attending, she discovered the *real* reason God had wanted her there . . . so she could be healed of a depression that she had been battling for a long time. She shared with me that the healing process began at the seminar. She was moved to seek out Christian counseling and for the first time in years was feeling a freedom from depression. I finally met her a few months later when she came to visit our church. She had a smile on her face and said that the healing was continuing![20]

Making the Right Connections between People

Because it is impossible for the parish nurse to be the only one who can make situations better, it is essential that the nurse become a multiplier of people and resources. Just as it is important for the nurse to assess what is needed in a given situation, it is important for the nurse to make the right connections between and among people so that healing occurs. Carole Kornelis knew the right connection.

JUST RECENTLY I received a phone call from one of our young church members, who needed help with a distraught friend who had recently lost her husband. This friend is very new in her faith; she felt that life was unfair and that God was silent when she prayed. I linked her to someone who understood grief and loss and had much compassion and love to offer. This young woman called to thank me for connecting her with someone who really understood. She also said that for the first time since her husband's death, she had slept well.

Anna Friedberg shares another example of being a good "matchmaker."

I WILL NEVER FORGET when one of our church members was ill and unable to manage the housework. I knew of another church member who is learning disabled but is certainly able to do housework. I paired them up and it turned out even better than I anticipated. I thought only that I was getting housework done for the one woman, but I guess God had other plans. The woman who was ill was assisted with her housework. However, the learning disabled woman loved to hear Bible stories read out loud, so the woman who was ill read Scripture and helped the learning disabled woman with her reading skills as well!

Bringing Together a Community of Healing and Love

The last story of joy is shared by Kristine Holmes. She describes how a community came together for healing and love.

IN THE SUMMER of 2000 a young couple returned to our church family after a brief time away. The wife informed me that after experiencing numerous miscarriages she was finally pregnant. Later in the month she told me that they were expecting triplets. We discussed resources available to them, including their own families, the church family, and organizations such as Moms of Multiples. I agreed to check her blood pressure each week as directed by her physician.

In early September she developed hypertension and was placed on bed rest. I coordinated a meeting of the Health Ministry Team, deacons, and women's associations to develop a plan to assist with meals and friendly visits. I continued to visit frequently to monitor her blood pressure. The members of the church's Prayer Tree lifted Mom and babies up in prayer. In late October she went into labor and was admitted to the hospital.

On November 3, Charlie, Carrie, and Katie were born by Cesarean section and each weighed in at slightly over two pounds. The congregation prayed mightily for these babies and their parents. Word spread to other congregations in the area as well as out of state and more prayers were offered for their health and safety.

Our associate pastor and I were allowed to visit the Neonatal Intensive Care Unit regularly. We prayed with the parents and with the hospital staff. I brought pictures of the babies to the church and placed them in my office window. This eventually became a visual growth chart that I updated with new pictures after every hospital visit. Members of the congregation made a point to walk by my office so they could check on the babies. We provided regular progress reports to the congregation during our church services and to the members of the Prayer Tree.

During one of my visits to an elderly (eighty-six-year-old) homebound woman, I told her about Charlie, Carrie, and Katie. Eagerly, she said that she would pray for them. Part of my weekly duties then included a phone call or visit to update her on the progress of the babies. She became their "prayer warrior."

Just before Christmas, Charlie came home. The deacons and women's associations continued to provide meals and assistance so that Mom could visit Carrie and Katie, both of whom remained in the hospital. Carrie came home in early January and

Katie, whose stay was lengthened because of two surgeries, came home at the end of January, on Super Bowl Sunday. How appropriate that the Baltimore Ravens won the game! Once again, I took a photo—this time with a Ravens blanket covering their car seats.

"Moms" of all ages pitched in to fold clothes, rock babies, wash dishes, and prepare meals. The babies' eighty-six-year-old prayer warrior continued to pray.

On Mother's Day, at six months of age, the triplets were baptized. I was privileged to assist during the service and I carried Charlie down the aisle to introduce him to his church family. As the pastor, a deacon, and I carried the children, members of the congregation reached out to touch them, as if to touch God's special work.

Two weeks after their baptism, I helped Mom load the babies into their van and we took them to see their prayer warrior—a wonderful woman who had faithfully held them in prayer. What a wonderful sight! Smiling babies and a woman whose heart overflowed with joy. *Those* pictures are in frames in my office.

Prayers, love, the helping hands of young and old, an entire community, helped strengthen this young family and our whole congregation. I am humbled to have witnessed God's abundant grace.

The stories of parish nurses recorded here tell us that parish nursing involves a call, a response of faith to that call, and an unending journey. Nurses have shared stories of challenge and joy that woven together form a tapestry of love, service, and dedication. In a very real sense, the journey is the destiny. In the next chapter, parish nurses share with us the ways in which God has taken their journeys beyond the church and into the community at large.

CHAPTER 4

The Journey into the Community

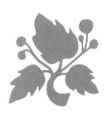

Journeys have a way of producing detours and side trips that are not part of the original itinerary. Most of us map out our path by identifying the most direct route and trying to avoid detours that add time or hazards to the trip. Our goal is to reach our destination. However, if indeed the journey is the destination, we may find unexpected joys when we wander off the beaten path, especially when those meanderings are not part of our planned agenda.

Most nurses involved in congregational health ministry plan a journey that focuses their energies on the needs of a specific church. As with any journey, preparation is required. The traveler needs to know what to pack; she needs to know about the terrain; she needs to know what personal resources are required; and she needs to know the expected time of arrival. As nurses reflect on whether or not they are called to parish nursing, they embark on a similar process of preparation. They pack their nursing knowledge and skills along with a deep commitment that they are responding to God's call. They take stock of the "lay of the land" of their own church, deciding whether the territory is friendly or hostile toward a health ministry. Beyond their nursing expertise they reflect on the personal resources that are required, such as infinite patience, excellent communication and negotiation skills, ability to work with groups, knowledge of Scripture and the faith statements of their own denomination, and the ability to draw the best from others. They engage in additional preparation for the journey through their reading about this new specialty and their enrollment in various parish nurse preparation courses. They are usually confident about where they are going on this journey, although they generally underestimate the time required to arrive at a destination point where parish nursing is firmly established in their congregations. These nurses are sometimes surprised to discover that God has other plans and the destination to which He calls them is beyond the walls of the congregation!

Scripture contains many stories about journeys that took unexpected twists and turns. God led the Israelites out of the familiar land of the Egyptians and allowed them to wander through the Sinai desert experiencing years of adventures, close calls, and unexpected opportunities. Just so He leads nurses from the familiar territory of hospital or community-based nursing into the new and uncharted lands of congregational nursing, to the previously unknown domains of educator of parish nurses and coordinator for networks of congregational health ministries, to the unmapped frontier of faith-based community nursing.

These forays beyond the individual church and into the community are an extension of what God calls nurses to do within the church—educate the unlearned, support those who are unsure, calm the anxious, feed the hungry, give drink to the thirsty, clothe the naked, house the homeless, provide rest to the weary, visit the lonely, care for the sick, and offer employment to the jobless. These needs exist in our churches, our neighborhoods, our cities, our country, and our world. The call of God is to take what He gives to us, and just as Jesus multiplied the fish and loaves to feed the five thousand, nurses are to multiply their individual resources to minister within churches and beyond. How has God called parish nurses beyond the confines of their churches? In this chapter we present five stories. The first tells how God called the nurse to minister to other parish nurses; the second focuses on God's call to develop health ministries within poor and underserved churches; the third relates how God called a nurse to extend her parish nursing into a community-based clinic to serve some of the poorest and neediest among His kingdom; the fourth and fifth describe how God has called nurses to reach out and embrace the needs of those who suffer from domestic violence.

A Journey of Ministry to Parish Nurses

Tom Pruski became the coordinator of a health ministry and parish nurse program called Wellness Works in October 1999. Wellness Works is a unique partnership between Catholic Charities of the Archdiocese of Washington, D.C., and the Montgomery County Health and the Human Services Department in Maryland. At the time Tom shared his story with us, he coordinated six partnering congregations of different faiths that were developing models of health ministry and parish nursing. In order to disseminate information about health ministry and local health ministry events, he taught himself website design and established a website.[1] Tom tells how he was led into coordinating and ministering to parish nurses.

MY CALL INTO NURSING took a circuitous route. After high school, I entered college as a psychology major. I was interested in people and how they interacted with the world around them. During my first year of college, my grandmother who lived with my family died of breast cancer. She was a quiet soul who spoke with humility and grace. Her presence had a great effect on my upbringing and my concept of family. While I was still in high school, she had been paralyzed on one side of her body as a result of a series of strokes. My parents had decided to make her a permanent part of our family and she moved in with us. This decision had a huge impact on my life as well as on the lives of my siblings. We all participated in her care, including her physical care. We helped to brush her teeth and walked her to the bathroom. Despite her physical disabilities she had a good sense of humor that kept everyone lighthearted and at ease. With her death, I began to think seriously about reconsidering my college career goals and plans.

During the summer of my senior year in high school, my older brother decided to become a nursing assistant at a local nursing home. Through his experience I got my first exposure to the profession of nursing. He told me stories about the residents and how they appreciated him being there. At that time, he was the only male nursing assistant and he talked about the challenge of that situation. He also shared with me the rewards of his patient care and interactions with the residents. He left after the summer to enter college and pursue a degree in pharmacology. After my grandmother died, I thought a lot about the time I had spent caring for her. I thought a lot about the stories my brother had told me. Following my freshman year in college and my summer break, I decided to try my hand at nursing and I became a nursing assistant.

Indeed, nursing home work was hard. Just like my brother before me, I was the only male on the nursing staff. At times, being the only male was lonely. Although the work was physically exhausting, there were inspirational moments where I was privileged to comfort a dying patient, to receive birthday cards from patients, and to learn the life stories of many of the residents. This experience, combined with the death of my grandmother, influenced my decision to become a nurse. I wanted my career choice to affirm my desire to become a more caring and compassionate person. Nursing provided that environment and opportunity. I changed my major to nursing and I graduated from Niagara University with a bachelor's degree in nursing.

After nursing school, I worked at Strong Memorial Hospital on a neuro-gero psychiatric unit in Rochester, New York. I remember many of my professors telling me to go to a medical-surgical unit in order to reinforce my basic medical-surgical skills. However, I wanted to work in an environment that encouraged care of the body as well as the mind and spirit. Initially, I found such a work environment at Strong on this special nursing unit. I knew it would be challenging and demanding and it was, especially to a new graduate. Sad to say the hospital environment did not live up to my expectations. After a year, I felt burned out and needed a break. I believed that I was being called to a different place.

I spent time reflecting and praying. Back in college I had heard about a volunteer corps called the Vincentian Service Corp-East, an organization sponsored by the Vincentians that provided year-long volunteer experiences in three inner cities. Volunteers lived in community with each other in New York, Philadelphia, or Washington, D.C. One day at the hospital, I picked up the phone and called a friend of mine who was a Daughter of Charity, a religious sister. She gave me the name of the director of the Vincentian Service Corp-East. I called him and he remembered having met me at a college event. He told me that Christ House, a medical facility for homeless men in Washington, D.C., needed a volunteer nurse for a year. Then he called Christ House and they asked if I could fly down for an interview. I flew down that weekend and they offered me the job if I wanted it.

I told them that I had to pray about my decision. They were very supportive. I prayed and felt that God was calling me to this new challenge. I believed that this was an opportunity to grow and to experience new things. I let them know I was taking the job. Little did I realize how much this decision would change my life's journey!

My volunteer year helped me to see a new perspective on life. Living in community with people from different backgrounds taught me a lot about others and myself. In fact, I still keep in touch with many of the people I met. My experience at Christ House taught me more than I can tell you. I learned to break down my own stereotypes. I learned to know the names and stories of homeless men with whom I worked. They taught me a great deal about patience and humility.

After my volunteer year, I prayed again about where God wanted me to go next. I decided to go to seminary to study theology and to discern if the priesthood was where God was calling me. I had thought about the priesthood before, but this seemed like a natural direction to go after my fulfilling volunteer year.

After a year in seminary, I decided that the priesthood was not where God was calling me. However, I still wanted to continue to study theology as a lay student. I found work as a nurse at a psychiatric facility for men and women religious called St. Luke's Institute. St. Luke's mission appealed to me. It believes in an integrative approach of caring for the mind, body, and spirit. It is also one of the few places in the United States as well as the world that cares for religious men and women with this approach.

One of my friends in seminary asked me what I was interested in doing once I finished my studies in theology. I told him about my desire to find a place in nursing where I could provide whole person care, how I wanted to enhance my experience of work and community that I had felt at Christ House. He mentioned to me that he had a friend who was developing parish nursing in the area and that he understood that parish nursing focused on caring for the whole person. He put me in contact with his friend, Jeanne Nist, who was a parish nurse at Christ Lutheran Church in Silver Spring, Maryland. She introduced me to her role as a parish nurse and we quickly became friends.

As I completed my studies in theology school and worked at St. Luke's Institute, I began to see the connection between my theological study and my professional development as a nurse. I started to think more and more about parish nursing. I began to think about how parish nursing reaffirmed who I am and who I wanted to be. I felt like parish nursing was where God had been calling me for my whole life. After attending some of the regular networking meetings on parish nursing at Holy Cross Hospital in Maryland, I sensed a confirmation that this indeed was to be the next step in my journey. I felt like my place in the vineyard had finally been confirmed. I was at peace.

After graduating from Washington Theological Union in Washington, D.C., with a master of arts in pastoral studies, I began to look for employment opportunities in parish nursing. Parish nursing was still a fairly new concept and very few nurses even had volunteer positions in the Washington area. One day while working at St. Luke's Institute, I received a telephone call from Monsignor Ralph Kueher, the secretary of Social Concerns from the Archdiocese of Washington. He told me that the Archdiocese was interested in developing a parish nurse program and he wondered if I would be interested in heading up this project. Jeanne Nist had recommended me. I felt so thankful and joyful. I praised God for this wonderful opportunity and for leading my journey to this point. I accepted the position and my work in parish nursing began. Parish nursing ties together personal and professional experiences for me. I believe that God prepared me well for my role. I continue to pray to God to provide guidance to me and all those with whom I work as coordinator of parish nursing and health ministries programs. I hope that through my parish nursing work I can both invite people to join and support others in this ministry.

Journey to Develop Lay Ministry Programs

Dr. Ruth Stoll's journey has taken her through many roles within parish nursing. She began as a teacher of parish nursing in the early 1990s and moved into an unpaid parish nurse position in her own church. Later, after retiring from teaching at Messiah College, she assumed a part-time paid parish nurse position at St. Stephen's Episcopal Cathedral in Harrisburg, Pennsylvania. After this her journey led out of the church into the development of lay ministry programs within African-American churches.

I WAS WORKING as a parish nurse at St. Stephen's Episcopal Cathedral in Harrisburg, Pennsylvania. I had been in the role for four years. Once the role of parish nurse was fully accepted and established within the congregation, I felt the Lord leading me beyond St. Stephen's. At first I was drawn to look into the Children's Checkup Center (CCC)—an outreach that St. Stephen's already had in place. The CCC was located in a public housing complex, called Hall Manor, that included five hundred apartments. I learned quickly that although there was outreach to the children residing in Hall Manor, there was nothing comparable for the adults—many of them single mothers. I spoke to the executive director of CCC about the possibility of conducting a door-to-door survey of the residents of Hall Manor, who were primarily of African-American and Latino descent. I received support from the church to do this as well. A Latino outreach worker and I offered free blood pressure screenings and administered a questionnaire to determine health risks as well as to discover whether or not these persons attended church and if there was anything other than worship that their churches offered. I discovered that most of the residents didn't attend church with any regularity, and their churches offered little beyond worship and church school. I also discovered that there were many "store front" churches in the area but neither these small churches nor the larger, more established denominations were reaching significantly into this community. Health ministry was nonexistent; few of these churches had members who were health professionals.

As I became increasingly aware of the vast unmet spiritual, physical, and emotional needs, I felt God calling me to do something about it. I resigned my position as part-time parish nurse at

St. Stephen's and committed myself to the development of lay models of health ministry within the African-American and Latino congregations. Initially, I made some overtures to the Latino churches in the area but discovered that they were not receptive at that time.

So I started to focus my attention on the African-American churches. I met a young African-American man in the legal aid society in Harrisburg who offered to help me make contact with three African-American congregations. He suggested that I needed to come to the churches with something to offer them, something similar to an AIDS prevention program that had recently been offered to this same community. I did some exploration into the AIDS prevention program as well as other potential support resources. I went to the Penn State Extension Agency and presented my idea for a 22.5 hour certificate program designed to develop lay health facilitators prepared to start health ministries within African-American churches. My proposal was approved. Initially, my efforts focused on the three congregations where I had already made contact.

The program that I presented at the three churches covered five major topics. The first was on healthy lifestyles including diet and exercise. Under this topic I was able to use some videos relevant to the African-American population. One video dealt with decreasing fat in the diet and another dealt with alternatives to frying food that still produced tasty and nutritious meals. The second topic, high-risk concerns of the population, included training the participants to take blood pressure readings on themselves and others. The focus was on the prevention of hypertension and heart disease. The third topic focused on diabetes prevention and complications. The fourth dealt with depression and anxiety. The fifth and last topic focused on how to use this information within the congregation to start a health ministry. These five topics were covered in nine classes.

In the first church, eight participants completed the entire program and earned the certificate. There were twice that number who attended individual classes but chose not to complete the entire program. Similar results occurred in the other churches. Six completed the program in the second church. Seven completed the nine-session course in the third church. I also offered CPR certification and two of the churches took advantage of this opportunity. An additional session, for one of the churches, dealt with health directives, the importance of organizing personal papers, and making decisions about health-care wishes. Throughout the classes I wove a strong spiritual and scriptural base. We began every class with prayer and usually one of the participants assumed responsibility for leading the worship aspect of the class.

Right now we are working to establish the role of health facilitator. One of the churches is very independent and I am serving mostly as a cheerleader and consultant. The other two churches require me to assume a more active role. My ultimate goal is that they will all be independent with fully functioning health ministries. I have evaluated the programs and found that most of the participants suggested very minor changes and reported that they had experienced changes in their attitudes toward healthy living and an increase in exercise!

To get one of the churches started financially, I wrote a grant proposal and submitted it to the Central Pennsylvania Episcopal Diocese; I received a two thousand dollar grant that came with the promise of another one thousand dollars if I could obtain a matching grant for a thousand dollars. I was able to obtain the matching grant. I plan to approach the Greater Harrisburg Foundation for a similar grant for the second church.

When I look back to 1990 when I first became involved in the parish nurse movement, I see how the Lord has led me increasingly to broaden my perspective. First, as a faculty member at Messiah College, I focused on individual nurses and prepared them to function within congregations. Later, I realized the importance of creating a network of support for parish nurses and began an annual parish nurse conference held at Messiah College that drew over one hundred nurses every year. My next move was into the role of parish nurse for St. Stephen's, where the Lord allowed me not only to minister to the congregation but also to see how my skills as a parish nurse and a parish nurse educator could benefit a poor and underserved community. It has certainly been an exciting journey.[2]

Journey to Minister to the Poor and Underserved

Maggie Spielman held a parish nurse position at Swedish Covenant Hospital in Chicago when she heard that the hospital was looking for ways to extend its parish nurse program to serve the inner city poor. Maggie explored this opportunity and became the first parish nurse in a homeless shelter on the North Side of Chicago. The shelter is called Cornerstone Community Outreach and is run by The Jesus People USA (JPUSA), a part of the Evangelical Covenant denomination. The Jesus People view the shelter as an extension of their church family and treat it as such. Maggie's story has two important components: her conversion to Christianity and her journey into faith-based community parish nursing.

I WAS A CERTIFIED transcultural nurse and really into this cultural thing. I was drawn to applied anthropology, one of the disciplines foundational to transcultural nursing. I believed that God and values were relative to whatever culture you came from, and as a nurse I wanted to preserve cultures. I wanted to reinforce traditional cultural beliefs. At that time, I was opposed to missionaries because I felt they destroyed cultures. I was entrenched in New Age thinking and cultural relativism. Then I met Jesus and slowly over the next few years my worldview completely changed. I . . . realized that the role of the nurse in the shelter environment could encompass all the things a parish nurse does in the more traditional setting of the church: integrator of faith and health, health educator, personal health counselor, liaison with congregational and community resources, and health advocate.

Looking back, I now know that I wasn't a Christian when I took the position, although I believed I was. My hook was the culture. I wanted to study and understand homelessness as a subculture and then provide culturally congruent care. The Jesus People did not ask me what my beliefs were when I interviewed for the position. They may have assumed mine were the same as theirs. They just saw that I wanted to work with homeless people and that I'd done it in the past. They believe that God sends them people who need to be there, and I needed to be there. I thought the job would be interesting and cultural, and that's all I wanted. But then, over time, my friends at Jesus People shared the gospel with me, mostly through how they lived their lives and interacted with the homeless people placed in their care.

At about the same time, another parish nurse invited me to a Bible Study Fellowship group, and that's when I realized that something was missing in my life. One day the teaching leader said that we could pray a prayer of assurance, so I went home and told God I wasn't sure and I wanted to be sure. I wanted to have a relationship with God through Jesus Christ. Through their actions, my friends had opened my eyes to how authentic Christians live and behave. I became a believer because I saw it lived!

This is an amazing place to work because the staff has great fellowship, and we pray with and for our clients. Since I came here, I have never had anyone say "no" to prayer. The shelter draws people from all over the city and it is always full. Eighty to ninety people are in the shelter at all times, and I know every one of them.

When I come through the door, they start telling me their health woes. We prefer that they come through the centralized system because the Department of Human Services tracks people who are homeless. However, we have taken people who just show up, but we prefer not to do that.

One day recently, a couple came to the shelter. The woman was in renal failure—a diabetic on dialysis. We were full, but we made room. The only spot to be found was a storage area. We had been hoping to turn it into a lounge, but we moved everything out and put in some cots, and that's where they're staying. The wife is scheduled for heart surgery next week, and I have had the opportunity to pray with her about that. My routine changes dramatically when we have someone like this show up. My focus will be on the woman and her husband for a while because I will act as the case manager for them.

Another time we had a mother with developmental delays who had several children with hernias. In the past she had been unable to schedule and coordinate the presurgical work-up for the children. We knew that she couldn't handle this situation on her own, so we made it a priority to get the surgeries completed while she lived at the shelter so we could help her.

Emergencies are not uncommon at the shelter. Sue, my Bible study leader, is good at making practical applications of what we are studying. One day she said that rather than come to the Lord with an agenda, we should say, "Show me what you have for me today." I remember distinctly the day I prayed that prayer. I was conducting a class with the moms, and they had their kids with them because the day care was full. A new woman came into the group, with her baby wrapped in layers of blankets. He was extremely quiet, but it didn't really concern me.

Near the end of the class we were discussing some aspect of HIV, when the woman with the baby said in a timid voice, "Oh, my baby's been sick, but . . ." And then someone else interrupted her and started talking. When the class ended, everyone needed something. I got so involved with these other concerns that the woman and her baby just disappeared. Something whispered to me (I'm sure it was the Holy Spirit) and said, "You've got to go find that baby."

I went upstairs to the dormitory and found the woman and the baby. After unwrapping the mass of blankets, I took one look at him and knew he was severely dehydrated. We rushed him to Children's Memorial Hospital, and he was admitted for ten days. He could have died! I remember how inundated I'd been that day, with people saying, "Do this" and "Do that." But this quiet, little voice told me to follow up with this woman—a life was saved. That was the Lord.

If you're in this work to help people change and expect to see that change while they're here, you'll be disappointed. But we have a heart for the people we are serving, and that seems unique to this shelter. Love makes the difference. Love is the key. Many women who come here have never been loved and, in fact, they have suffered a lot of abuse. They are surrounded by love here. They'll always be able to look back and say that they were cared for by people who were concerned about them as individuals made in the image of God. That's what parish nursing is all about.[3]

Journey to Minister to the Abused and Wounded

Kristine Holmes is active as a full-time parish nurse for First Presbyterian Church in Howard County, Maryland. However, in the last few years the Lord has extended her journey as well. Although her focus remains her congregation, she has reached out to embrace the surrounding community in several ways.

WHEN I BEGAN to make our congregation aware of the extent of domestic violence and our responsibility as a caring community I had the full support of the pastor and associate pastor as well as the health ministry team. I placed information posters in each stall of the women's bathroom. The information posters included tear-off sheets on what steps to take in leaving an abuser, what precautions to take, what numbers to call, and so on. Within a few days of my posting this information, every tear-off sheet was gone! Needless to say I was surprised. I couldn't believe or maybe I didn't want to believe that there could be that much need for this information within my congregation. By the end of the next week, again all of the tear-off sheets were gone.

Then it dawned on me that our church facility is used by many groups within the community and I felt the Lord nudge me to begin an outreach to these organizations. I contacted the Domestic Violence Center of Howard County, STAR (Sexual Treatment, Advocacy, and Recovery) Center for victims of sexual trauma, and the sheriff's department. I discovered that each of the facilities had different needs that I thought that we as a congregation could meet.

The Domestic Violence Center of Howard County identified a need for paper products, cleaning supplies, sanitary supplies for women, soap, shampoo, hair conditioner, and body lotion. The STAR Center expressed a need for clean sets of clothing. Many times when sexually traumatized women are treated at a hospital, their clothes are taken as evidence by the police. Even when the clothes are not confiscated by the police, the women don't want to wear the clothes that they had on when they were attacked. The clothing evokes painful memories and makes them feel unclean. As a result, the women have no clothing to wear out of the hospital. The STAR Center specifically requested sets of underwear, sneakers, and jogging suits. I took these requests back to our church and several of the women's groups have taken this up as their mission. They bring these supplies to my office every week and I make sure they get to the shelters. In fact, I have a basket in my office where church members drop samples of soaps, shampoos, conditioners, lotions, and other toiletries that they pick up at hotels. I then pass these on to one of the shelters.

The sheriff's office has a program to collect unused mobile phones. They take responsibility for getting batteries for the telephones and getting the phones charged. Even though the phone is not connected, a call to 911 is always possible as long as the phone is charged. The sheriff's office then distributes these phones to women and to seniors who might need to make an emergency telephone call. Again my congregation has assumed this as another ministry project and on a regular basis I deliver unused cell phones to the sheriff's office.

In the last year I have been involved in coordinating the parish nurse/health ministry efforts in Howard County. As part of this role, I have made sure that each of the nurses from participating congregations receives the posters and information cards related to domestic violence. Many of these nurses are also participating in the collection of used cell phones. During one of our network meetings, I arranged for a representative from the Domestic Violence Center to speak to the nurses and we watched the video *Broken Vows,* which looks at the problem of domestic violence from the perspective of different faith traditions.[4]

Terrill Stumpf's journey has taken him through many twists and turns, including serving as a parish nurse at Old First Presbyterian Church in San Francisco. At present he is the director of Health Ministry at Fourth Presbyterian Church in Chicago. Terry serves on the leadership teams of the Presbyterian Parish Nurse Task Force as well as the Presbyterians Against Domestic Violence Network, which is part of the Presbyterian Health, Education, and Welfare Association of the Presbyterian Church (U.S.A.). Each of these positions extends the focus of his nursing journey beyond the church.

For instance, at Old First Presbyterian he worked at a senior activity center. In his leadership roles in the Presbyterian Church, God has called Terry to serve and educate other parish nurses and to reach out to women who are trapped in abusive situations. His journey has taken him into domestic violence prevention.

I DEVELOPED a worship service focusing not only on the effects of domestic violence, but also on God's response to the pain, suffering, brokenness, and frequent death that results from domestic violence. I emphasized that God's intention for the world is that we do no wrong and commit no acts of violence against one another. The worship service is intended to encourage participants to lift up the silent voices of those who live daily in fear or in actual violence to themselves and their children. Because of the intense emotional tone of the worship service, some in attendance experienced strong psychological responses and felt the need to talk to someone during or following the service. I made sure that this support service was provided. Participants were encouraged to light a candle for someone they hold in their hearts who is or has been touched by domestic violence. The worship service was structured to include a combination of relevant Scripture readings, musical selections, a secular reading, prayers for healing, a unison prayer, a recitation of the Lord's Prayer, and finally dismissal. The visual background for the service was created using a display of t-shirts and a memory quilt obtained from the Clothesline Project in Chicago.[5] This display gives witness to the violence against women. The quilt includes the names of women who have died because of domestic violence. The t-shirts hung around the room include white t-shirts for women who have died of violence; yellow or beige for women who have been battered or assaulted; red, pink, or orange for women who have been raped or sexually assaulted; blue or green for women who are survivors of incest or child sexual abuse; and purple or lavender for women attacked because of their sexual orientation. In addition to the visual display, playing softly in the background is the "Sounds of Silence," also created by the Clothesline Project. These sounds include a gong that is struck every ten seconds to acknowledge the battering of a woman that occurs every ten seconds in the United States; a whistle that is blown every one minute to mark the rape of a woman every one minute in the United States; and a bell that tolls every fifteen minutes to acknowledge the deaths of four women who are killed daily by men who supposedly loved them.

One morning I offered this worship as the morning prayer service at Fourth Presbyterian Church where I am the director of health ministries. The invitation to worship is extended to the community at large as well as the staff and congregation of the church. Among the participants was a woman who is a member of the church. I could see that the service had a tremendous emotional impact on her although she did not leave the service or seek individual counsel. Later in the day she came to my office and shared that the service had not only opened up wounds that she thought were healed, but also brought necessary healing to these buried wounds. Throughout the service she was flooded with vivid memories of her mother's abuse at the hands of her father and then later in life, her own abuse at the hands of her first husband. We talked and prayed together and she expressed a peace that she had not felt in a very long time. I am thankful how God has taken me on a journey that leads to healing, reconciliation, and wholeness—both within the church congregation and beyond.[6]

The stories of these nurses are a reminder of God's depth and breadth. His call to nurses is not limited to a particular church or congregation. He calls nurses to be yeast and light to a broken world—yeast to multiply and expand works of compassion, concern, and care certainly both within and beyond congregational walls, and light to illuminate the needs that are there to be met, the talents of people who can meet these needs, and the paths to be taken. In the refrain of a hymn by Rory Cooney entitled "Jerusalem, My Destiny," Cooney aptly captures the sentiment of a journey led by God. "I have fixed my eyes on your hills. Jerusalem, my destiny! Though I cannot see the end for me, I cannot turn away. We have set our hearts for the way; this journey is our destiny. Let no one walk alone. The journey makes us one."[7]

Thus far we have focused on how God calls nurses and their response to His call as He leads them on a journey to parish nursing and beyond. In the next chapter we shift our attention to the preparation needed for these journeys. It is said that God does not necessarily call those who are prepared but that He prepares those whom He calls. In the next chapter, we will examine the ways in which God prepares parish nurses.

CHAPTER 5

Preparation for the Journey

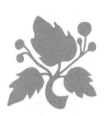

Most people embarking on a new journey seek advice from others who have taken a similar path. Commencement exercises traditionally feature speakers who point graduates in the direction of fulfillment. Anna Quindlen, a Pulitzer Prize-winning columnist, wrote a commencement speech for the graduates of Villanova University. Although she never gave the speech, it was published as *A Short Guide to a Happy Life* and earned a long-standing place on the *New York Times* bestseller list.[1] The phenomenal success of this book gives a glimpse into our longing for mentors and guides. Quindlen reminds readers that life is limited, that we need to make the most of it and devote ourselves to meaningful activities.

Another enormously successful book, *Tuesdays with Morrie,* provides the reader with the insights of Morrie Schwartz, a sociology professor who was dying of ALS.[2] Morrie's shared wisdom focused on death, fear, greed, society, forgiveness, and a meaningful life. Schwartz noted, "People see me as a bridge, I'm not as alive as I used to be, but I'm not dead yet . . . I'm on the last great journey here—and people want me to tell them what to pack."

This quest for mentors and guides derives from a rich religious heritage. Ancient Hebrews believed that living a good and happy life in community with neighbor and God was something that could be learned. Proverbs, psalms, and stories were used to teach successive generations of Israel's children the secrets of a rewarding life.[3] Today many still look to Scripture for wisdom, guidance, and truths that can aid us in making life both more meaningful and more manageable.

Nurses who embark on the journey into parish nursing have already taken the advice of Quindlen, Schwartz, and countless biblical writers who point us away from a focus on the self to a focus on the other. Who are the mentors for parish nurses? Who are the adventurers who share their wisdom to light the parish nurse journey? How does God prepare the nurses who are called to parish nursing? These questions are answered by examining the roots of the parish nurse movement and by exploring how those roots have expanded and evolved since 1984 when the Reverend Granger Westberg formalized the concept of parish nursing. Westberg led the way, but he forged a path that has been further cleared by countless other nurse leaders. This chapter looks at several of these leaders and the contributions they have each made to parish nurse preparation.

The Reverend Granger Westberg

In an interview published in the 1989 issue of the *Journal of Christian Nursing,* Westberg traced the beginnings of the parish nurse concept to an experience he had as a pastor of a church in Illinois in 1940.

> ONE DAY at a Lutheran pastors' conference in Chicago, several other young ministers and I sat with the seventy-seven-year-old chaplain of Augustana Lutheran Hospital. In the course of our conversation, this chaplain explained that he needed to be away from the hospital for a week. "Would one of you fellows like to take my place?" he asked. "I'd like to do that," I said. "I think it would be fun." That was the beginning of one of the greatest weeks of my life.
>
> I was able to minister to patients effectively in a very short time. When people are lying horizontally in a hospital, they begin to think about the vertical dimension of life. They wonder about the meaning of life and start asking spiritual questions. But

there's usually no one around to help them deal with those difficult questions, so they don't get very far with their thinking.

All during that life-changing week I came in contact with
people who needed help to think deeply and productively. I
hope I helped them, as I injected biblical concepts into their
thinking.

Just over three years later, as a result of contacts made that
week, I became the chaplain at Augustana. That was 1944. I was
thirty years old then, and people were just beginning to see the
potential for changing lives through hospital ministry.

Over the years, ministering and teaching at Augustana and
then at the University of Chicago, I began to see that a person's
physical well-being was tied to his or her emotional and spiritual
health. Again and again as I talked to patients, I found that their
illnesses seemed to originate in some personal struggle, often related to grief.

I felt that the key to preventive medicine lay in picking up
people's early cries for help. Someone needed to be on the scene
in the church to deal with people before they became seriously
ill.[4]

From these understandings, Westberg developed a wholistic
health center to provide health care in a poor community.

WE OPENED up a free clinic in a church, signed up two volunteer doctors and one volunteer nurse and used seminary students
to do counseling. Subsequently, we set up clinics in middle- and
upper-income communities where people paid standard fees for
the services. A nurse, doctor, and pastor would treat these people's
complaints wholistically, recognizing that their problems stemmed
from and affected not only the body, but also the mind and spirit.

But these clinics were expensive to start and operate. We had
to pay the salaries of three or four professionals and the cost of
renovating a building. And we had to subsidize operations be-

cause we couldn't charge a high-enough fee to cover the expense of treatment by three people instead of just one. However, a dozen of these clinics are still in operation across the country.

I realized that the nurse was the key member of the professional team in these clinics. (So far all of them have been women.) She had the sensitivity—the peripheral vision, I call it—to see beyond the patient's problems and verbal statements. She could hear things that were left unsaid. And she was the best listener.

For example, when we would conduct initial interviews with patients, it was the nurse who really heard what was said. Then afterward she would give feedback to the doctor and the pastor. "Do you remember when Mrs. Olson was starting to tell you something, and you butted in and gave a little sermonette, Doctor (or Pastor)? She had something important to say, I think, and you stopped her."

Nurses seem to have one foot in the sciences and one in the humanities, one foot in the spiritual world and one in the physical world. The nurses I've had the privilege to work with have been very perceptive; they have great insight into the human condition.

So many nurses I work with have a deep spiritual desire to help people. They don't view the hospital as a warehouse for sick bodies. They see people as sacred in God's eyes. Consequently, they look at the whole person, not just the ailment.

When many doctors enter a patient's room, too often they view the patient with a sort of tunnel vision. They see the physical problem and nothing else. If the patient has something wrong with his or her arm, doctors will go right to the arm, take care of it and leave. Maybe they spend only a few minutes with that person. In many cases they say almost nothing to the patient beyond asking about physical symptoms.

But nurses entering the same room will see and hear a great

deal more than some doctors. Nurses may comment on pictures or get-well cards, or talk with family members who've come to visit—all at the same time that they are caring for the patient's physical needs.

One day, while lamenting the expense of running a wholistic health center, a friend said, "You keep saying such wonderful things about nurses. Instead of opening a clinic, what if we just put a nurse on the church staff? Would that work?"

We tried it, and it worked. Then I approached the president of Lutheran General Hospital in Park Ridge, Illinois, an old friend of mine. We discussed the concept of the parish nurse as a practitioner in preventive health care. He was as excited about it as I was. So we decided to test out the idea in six Chicago-area churches—four Protestant and two Catholic.

The six churches each chose a nurse. We gave them a list of applicants, and the congregations also had women who were interested in the positions.

Lutheran General agreed to sponsor the program by paying 75 percent of the half-time salary for each nurse the first year. The second year the hospital paid 50 percent and 25 percent the third year. Thus each year Lutheran General paid less and the churches paid an increasing percentage of their nurse's salary. By the fourth year, each church was paying the nurse's full salary.

Each year, as the hospital reduced its contribution to the original six nurses, we added two more churches to the program with the extra money. Now we have over twelve.

Thus began the first parish nurse programs. But what about preparation? Was it enough to be a registered nurse or did Westberg find that additional preparation was required?

WE SET UP a low-key continuing education program at Lutheran General. Once a week the nurses met for half a day with me, the chaplains, a nurse from the hospital teaching program, and a doctor in family medicine. These people provided support and guidance for nurses.

When we got together the nurses shared stories about their ministry. Sometimes they role-played things that happened during the week. They exchanged ideas about ways to handle problems, and they had fellowship together and with the hospital chaplains.

When asked about the future of parish nursing, Westberg expressed a clear vision for this evolving nursing specialty.

I'D LIKE TO HAVE a thousand churches with parish nurse programs. We now have a Parish Nurse Resource Center at Lutheran General Hospital. I'd like to have a full-time director to run that. And, I'd like to see a special program for training parish nurses—either a six-week session at Lutheran General, or a staff member who would travel and train nurses on site.

Then I'd like to organize a parish nurse association to provide a newsletter and to set up local support groups for parish nurses. If I only had $35,000.

The Reverend Granger Westberg had a clear vision. He started the journey toward establishing parish nurses in individual churches and parish nursing as a new specialty—one that truly focuses on whole person health—physical, emotional, and spiritual. His vision and his wish list have all become realities. He took his vision and spoke across the country—to nursing groups, to nursing faculty teaching in Christian-based colleges and universities, and to hospital personnel. His mission was clear—to share the vision and to empower others to continue the journey he had begun.

Ann Solari-Twadell and the International Parish Nurse Resource Center

Unbeknownst to Westberg, God was orchestrating responses to Westberg's wish list across the entire country. Right in Westberg's backyard, Lutheran General Hospital hired Ann Solari Twadell to work on a pilot project called Congregational Health Partnership.[5] As Ann moved with uncertainty into her new role, she held onto the certainty that God had something important in mind. She was aware of this new concept of parish nursing. She knew that Westberg was sharing his vision nationwide and inspiring individuals to develop their own parish nursing programs. Ann was also aware that the original six parish nurses were being inundated with requests about "how to do it." The problem was that these requests were directed to nurses who were still in a pilot program themselves and were trying to discern the day-to-day operations of being parish nurses!

Ann recognized the need for resources and support for this growing movement. She went to her supervisor and proposed that Lutheran General establish a Parish Nurse Resource Center, which was endorsed in 1986. The center was formed out of the Office of Church Relations, Lutheran General Health Care System, in Park Ridge, Illinois. An advisory board was formed, with local and national nursing and clergy representation. It was this group that recommended that a membership group be formed separate and independent from the Resource Center. This suggestion led to the formation in September 1988 of the Health Ministries Association, a membership group made up largely of parish nurses but open to all types of health ministers.

In September 1987, the Parish Nurse Resource Center offered the first continuing education program on parish nursing. This initial offering evolved into the annual Westberg Symposium on Parish Nursing. This symposium offers pre-conference workshops on topics of current interest and features a nurse keynote speaker as well as a major clergy presenter. Abstracts for presentations and posters are solicited nationally and internationally. The conference includes worship, opportunities for networking, and produces a published book of proceedings that is distributed to all the participants. What began as a small local event drawing seventy-four participants in 1987 has grown to an international event with about one thousand participants from across the United States, Australia, Korea, Canada, England, and Ireland.[6]

In 1989, the Resource Center initiated a two and one-half day continuing education program called "Orientation to Parish Nursing." This program provided nurses with basic information regarding parish nursing, including how to get started, and a discussion of legal concerns and accountability. Included within the orientation was a half day of mentoring with one of the parish nurses sponsored by Lutheran General. This orientation program continued until 1996 when the Resource Center made a decision that initiation into parish nursing was best accomplished through "Basic Preparation," a lengthier and more in-depth program. The "Basic Preparation" course was developed from the input of nurses representing educational institutions across the United States as well as from regional parish nurse networks.

In 1995, Lutheran General Health Care System was purchased by Advocate Health Care System and the Parish Nurse Resource Center was renamed the International Parish Nurse Resource Center to reflect the expanding focus and influence of the center's work. Up until October 2001, the center continued its efforts to standardize parish nurse preparation, to study organizational models and functions, and to provide resources for the development of quality parish nurse programs through research, education, publishing, and consulting. When the center closed its doors in 2001, it had endorsed two standardized courses for parish nurses: the Basic Parish Nurse Preparation Course and the Parish Nurse Coordinator Course. Today there are approximately sixty providers across the country who meet the criteria established by the International Parish Nurse Resource Center to offer the curricula endorsed by the International Parish Nurse Resource Center. The content areas for each of these courses are detailed in Figures 5.1 and 5.2.

FIG 5.1. Core Curriculum Content for Basic Parish Nurse Preparation

- The Role of the Church in Health
- Theology of Health
- History of Parish Nursing
- Philosophy of Parish Nursing
- Models of Parish Nursing Practice
- Function of the Parish Nurse: Teacher
- Function of the Parish Nurse: Counselor
- Function of the Parish Nurse: Referral Agent
- Function of the Parish Nurse: Trainer of Volunteers
- Function of the Parish Nurse: Integrator of Faith and Health
- Community Assessment
- Health Promotion and Maintenance
- Faith Community and Family and Client
- Self-Care for the Parish Nurse
- Working with Churches
- Functioning within a Ministerial Team
- Accountability
- Documentation
- Legal Considerations
- Ethical Issues
- Prayer
- Worship Leadership
- Getting Started

FIG 5.2. Core Curriculum Content for Parish Nurse Coordinators

- The Role of the Parish Nurse Coordinator
- Working with Churches
- Trends in Healthcare
- Infrastructure for Parish Nurse Programs
- Accountability
- Documentation Systems
- Human Resource Management
- Budgeting
- Grant Writing
- Orientation of the New Parish Nurse
- Planning for the Ongoing Development of the Parish Nurse
- Continuing Education Experiential Sharing Exercise
- Spiritual Development of the Parish Nurse

Solari-Twadell, P. A., and McDermott, M. A., *Parish nursing: Promoting whole person health within faith communities,* p. 275, copyright © 1999. Reprinted by permission of Sage Publications, Inc.

Rosemarie Matheus and Marquette's Parish Nurse Preparation Institute

While Ann was developing the Parish Nurse Resource Center, God was raising up other parish nurses and parish nurse preparation programs. Rosemarie Matheus, director of the Parish Nurse Preparation Institute at Marquette University College of Nursing, had attended a church meeting where the first parish nurses from Illinois were speaking.[7] Rosemarie heard God speaking loud and clear to her during that meeting. She began to prepare a curriculum for parish nurses that was initially offered in 1990 at Concordia University in Mequon, Wisconsin. Nineteen nurses enrolled in Rosemarie's first class. This course was offered at Concordia for two years. Rosemarie then transferred the program to Marquette. In 1996, the Parish

Nurse Preparation Institute was established and Rosemarie became the director.

Dr. Norma Small and Dr. Ruth Stoll

Dr. Norma Small,[8] former associate dean for Graduate Studies and director of Gerontologic and Adult Health Nursing, School of Nursing, Georgetown University, Washington, D.C., and Dr. Ruth Stoll,[9] a former professor of psychiatric nursing at Messiah College in Grantham, Pennsylvania, represent two of the earliest forerunners in parish nurse preparation and each has a story to tell. Both Dr. Small and Dr. Stoll heard Westberg speak at Messiah College in 1988 and met with him. According to Dr. Small, the evolving role of the parish nurse called for an advanced practice nurse.

A YEAR AFTER my conversation with the Reverend Granger Westberg, I read his announcement in a Lutheran newsletter that Georgetown was beginning a parish nurse specialty in its master's program! I showed this announcement to the dean of the School of Nursing who gave me approval to develop and submit to the faculty a curriculum plan for parish health nursing as a new specialty in the graduate program. The faculty approved parish health nursing as a new specialty in 1989 and the first student was admitted in 1990. The program consisted of thirty-six hours of master's level courses. Twelve hours (three four-credit courses) were devoted to the specialty of parish nursing. These courses included the theory on health promotion, the integration of spirituality into wholistic nursing practice, and a parish nurse practicum. Students were encouraged to take electives in theology, spiritual direction, and courses related to their specific faith tradition. Georgetown developed an agreement with Washington Theological Union to open courses to graduate students in parish health nursing.

One of the major obstacles that Norma faced was finding a suitable site where students could complete the practicum in parish nursing.

> AT THAT TIME the closest parish nurse program was in Harrisburg, Pennsylvania—approximately a three-hour drive from Georgetown University. So I developed a parish nurse program at Christ Lutheran Church on 16th Street in Washington, D.C. I served the congregation for three years as a parish nurse while I provided mentoring for my students in their new roles. Three parish nurses graduated from this program. Unfortunately, Georgetown closed the program in 1993 because of the cost and the very limited market for master's prepared parish nurses.

Norma is retired from Georgetown but not from parish nursing. She continues to teach her own course for parish nurses and health ministers. The content of this curriculum differs from the curriculum endorsed by the International Parish Nurse Resource Center in that the content is derived from the *Scope and Standards of Parish Nursing Practice.*[10] Norma was part of the effort to develop this important document. The course is presented for thirty-five hours of continuing education credits in Johnstown, Pennsylvania. Every summer Norma also presents the course at Otterbein College in Columbus, Ohio. When the course is offered at Otterbein it is offered for both continuing education credits as well as for undergraduate and graduate credits. (See Appendix A for a copy of Norma's Concepts and Practice of Parish Nursing and Health Ministries curriculum.)

After Dr. Stoll heard Westberg speak at Messiah College she was also motivated to develop a course in parish nursing. Ruth describes her initial efforts in 1990 as a "stab in the dark"—there was so little concrete material to work with related to curriculum development.

> I WORKED with Jan Towers, another doctorally prepared nurse faculty member at Messiah. Our initial vision was that the course

would extend over a year and result in the awarding of a certificate in parish nurse practice. Through the end of 1991, thirteen students, Jan, and I met once every two weeks and the content focused equally on nursing and spiritual interventions.

Then I met Jo Sensenig, a parish nurse in a nearby Mennonite church. Jo had a master's in community health nursing and was very active in the Mennonite Health Ministry. As a result of my work with Jo, she and I revised the course so that we met every week in two evening workshops. This pattern continued for another year. Very quickly we decided that the course needed more time and structure. In 1992, we developed six continuing education courses based on what we believed were the key issues in parish nursing. In 1993, we began to teach these courses in evening and Saturday classes. Our first class of five nurses completed the courses and received a certificate of completion from Messiah College. We taught until the end of 1996 when Messiah decided to change its focus and no longer supported adult education efforts such as the parish nurse courses. A variety of individuals with a wide range of commitment to parish nursing and health ministry enrolled in the courses. Not all the students were interested in earning the certificate and not every student enrolled in the courses sequentially.

In addition to the certificate course that was offered at Messiah College, Ruth and Jo instituted an annual parish nurse conference. Conferences serve as another modality through which God prepares nurses who are called to parish nursing. Ruth describes the significance of these conferences.

EVEN MORE important than the course work that was developed and offered at Messiah was the parish nurse conferences that began in 1992 and continued until 1996. In 1992, the conference began as a one-day meeting with a keynote speaker, workshops, and opportunities for networking. By 1996, the conference had evolved into a two-day meeting held each June. Jo and I collaborated with Holy Spirit Hospital to sponsor the event. The impact of the conference was greater than we ever anticipated. By 1996, we had at least six hundred names on our mailing list with over one hundred people in attendance at the conference. The opportunities for networking and sharing of information were tremendous. Today, over six years later, nurses still tell me how valuable the conferences were!

Today Dr. Stoll is still actively involved in parish nurse education. At Lycoming College in Williamsport, Pennsylvania, she taught the elective courses for continuing education credits in parish nursing. Six nurses completed the courses for a certificate in parish nursing. She also teaches at Guthrie Health Care System in Sayre, Pennsylvania. Guthrie Health Care System is a provider approved by the International Parish Nurse Resource Center to offer the endorsed curriculum. Although the Guthrie program includes all the topics listed in Box 5.1, Ruth offers expanded content and hours of instruction to include more on spiritual foundation, theology of health and healing, spirituality and whole person health, integration of faith and health, values and ethics in health ministry, spiritual wholeness, and spiritual care. This expanded content is based on a scriptural understanding of health, healing, and wholeness. Today she is developing lay health ministries among African-American churches.

Carol Story and Puget Sound Parish Nurse Ministries

Carol Story, the Director of Puget Sound Parish Nurse Ministries, is another leader in parish nurse preparation.[11]

MY STORY BEGINS with simply becoming a nurse. Little did I know that every step in my career would lead me to become a parish nurse educator and program coordinator for a ministry. As I review my career, from my first job in the hospital working with all female patients, to being a supervisor in surgery, to office nursing, and even being an information and assistance worker for Senior Services, I can see how God has graciously led me though it all to be in this place at this time in my life. And I love it! I didn't become a Christian until I was thirty-two years old! He does work in mysterious ways.

My adventure in parish nursing began in 1992 when I attended a one-week intensive parish nurse class in Wisconsin. I came home excited and eager to begin a program in my church, but also with the thought of finding a means to begin an educational program for nurses who were interested in the concept. I continued to pray that God would give me direction and wisdom about where to go with the educational aspect that seemed to dominate my thoughts. I had not shared this with others because my reasoning was "who am I?" and "who would listen to me or take a class that I developed?" However, I had support and encouragement from my former dean, who had engaged another student and me to research the concepts of parish nursing. Today, she still continues to be an encourager!

God truly pulled strings to get me into graduate school (my GRE scores were terribly inadequate—I am a lousy test taker!) where I decided to go into program development and community health. Interestingly, I stumbled into a situation that made it possible for me to do my thesis work on spirituality and spiritual need in what was a secular university. I had the privilege of meeting and talking with an author of this book, Verna Carson, while at a Nurses Christian Fellowship (NCF) conference in the summer of 1992 when I took the parish nurse class. She also encouraged me to do the thesis work on spirituality. This is what really hooked me on the concept of parish nursing. I had a very strong sense that if nurses were going to work in churches, it was imperative that they (and I) understand the concept of spiritual care, spiritual need, and appropriately sharing their faith—even in their own congregations. Later, this same conviction led me to take a unit of clinical pastoral education. This was a decision that really changed my life and my walk with the Lord.

Soon after completing graduate school, I was invited to attend a meeting with nurses interested in parish nursing. Some of these nurses had taken an introductory course. When the leader, Dr. Ken Bakken, asked for a volunteer to coordinate some future meetings for this group, I agreed to do so—if at least four others would also. I remember telling the Lord that I would be willing to do whatever he wanted to spread the word about parish nursing—anything except speak in front of groups! The five of us met on a regular basis and we spent most of the meetings in prayer. I met with potential speakers and one of them said, "Why don't you develop an educational course for parish nurses?" I looked at him with a blank stare and then shared how God had given me that very goal many months before. Then he said he would write the pastoral care section. He was sure that Dr. Bakken, who had published a book on wholeness and healing in the Christian tradition, would write the section on the theology of healing and health. Suddenly, our group had a purpose: to provide education and support for nurses interested in parish nursing!

We submitted the course to the Washington State Nurses Association and received approval for sixty-two continuing education units. We held our first class in September 1994. Later we were invited to affiliate with Pacific Lutheran University. This allowed us to offer participants the option of receiving college credits or continuing education units. About this time I read a publication from the Parish Nurse Resource Center that listed suggested content for parish nurse courses. I was delighted to discover that the research and groundwork that my friend and I had done in 1992 had paid off—we exceeded those recommendations with the content we were offering in our course. Today, we partner with the International Parish Nurse Resource Center in their continued effort to standardize content and criteria for entry into practice. We have ten faculty, each expert in the content that they teach, blending their knowledge with the concepts of parish nursing. The class is offered twice a year in Seattle and since 1998, twice a year in Bellingham. A total of 150 nurses have now completed the class. This may seem like a small number, but our data reveals that 95 percent of these nurses have supportive and viable programs in their churches. Given the fact that Washington is the least churched state in the union, this is a blessing!

As a novice teacher, it was by faith alone that I accepted an invitation to facilitate a parish nurse class for the Free Methodist Women's Ministries in June 1995. Now I have done three for them. Since then, I have been invited to facilitate classes in San Diego, Los Angeles, and Kailua, Hawaii. God provides wonderful guest faculty, dedicated participants, and inspiring examples of how His people work together to blend faith and health in their communities.

Since 1993, our small interest group of nurses has grown to become a 501(c)3 tax-exempt nonprofit corporation, Puget Sound Parish Nurse Ministries, with a ten-member board of directors. We publish a quarterly newsletter, hold two annual continuing education conferences a year, and offer Parish Nurse Professional Development meetings in four different locations around Puget Sound. Many members, parish nurses, and supporters now speak publicly about parish nursing at annual conferences, within their denominations, and other churches; mentor nursing students interested in parish nursing; conduct research projects; write grants; and publish articles about parish nursing in local newspapers.

There is no greater honor than having women and men from multiple denominations come together to discover not only that they have much more in common then they have differences, but that God is really in *all* those churches, and that they can laugh, cry, and pray together and become one in God. Through parish nursing and involvement and membership in Health Ministries Association, I have had the privilege of meeting many people across the United States who are committed to the faith and health movement, to restoring the church's mission of healing. I am honored to be one small part of this movement.

The Reverend Sandra Thomas and Dr. Ruth Bell: Partners in Parish Nursing

The Reverend Sandra Thomas, the director of Partners in Parish Nursing, a Baltimore-based parish nurse preparation course, tells the story of this program.[12]

PARTNERS IN PARISH NURSING was formed in 1995 by a group of nine professionals in nursing and ministry. The group included Dr. Ruth Bell, a former faculty member from the University of Maryland School of Nursing, parish nurses, nursing educators, clergy, chaplains, pastoral counselors, and me. We came together seeking to develop an educational program in parish nursing that was congregationally based, had theological integrity, and included some spiritual formation experiences for students.

We developed a curriculum that integrates theological and nursing concepts into every module. It is based in systems theory and much attention is given to overlapping "systems" at work in caring relationships with individuals, families, congregation, and community.

With all the chaos and confusion in the world of education of parish nursing, and after "testing" the curriculum, we decided that parish nursing education needed to be at a graduate level. We all believed that parish nursing education should result in academic credit being granted—and should occur within the context of a theological school or graduate school of nursing. Thus, our current mission of providing the course in partnership with graduate schools began.

It is a rich and joyful process. The fact that the course takes place over time allows us to see the students wrestle with issues and grow. It is a most rewarding type of teaching and learning.

My dream is that more theological schools will come to see parish nursing as a new lay ministry and offer preparation cours-es—either ours or others.

One of our sites is at a state university—George Mason University School of Nursing and Health Sciences. We were able to "pass" the criteria for separation of church and state because we teach general theological concepts and assign the students to learn about their own specific denomination or religious affiliation. We provide resources and challenge them to learn and to be faithful to the professions of ministry in their churches and synagogues *and* to the profession of nursing.

(See Appendix A for Partners in Parish Nursing curriculum.)

The Reverend Donna Coffman and Caring Congregations

The Reverend Donna Coffman is the executive director for Caring Congregations, an associated program of Union Theological Seminary and Presbyterian School of Christian Education in Richmond, Virginia.[13] Coffman is also involved in parish nurse preparation and the curriculum that she offers is unique.

IN 1996, I attended an eight-day parish nurse preparation course taught by Rosemarie Matheus at Marquette University. When I returned home I reflected on the model of preparation that I had received and after discussing it with my partner at Union Theological Seminary, Dr. Henry Simmons, we developed a different model of preparation. I felt that what I had received was more of a "production model of preparation"—that it was designed to prepare me and others for the job of parish nursing. I envisioned a model that sees parish nursing as a spiritual journey rather than a job, focusing more on the spiritual development of nurses. This spiritual journey centers on learning to care for oneself so that offering care is a joy not a burden. With the help of Dr. Simmons I began to develop my ideas into a curriculum.

A friend of mine suggested that I meet with Carolyn Cuthrell, the community services manager for Health Corporation of America (HCA). HCA owns five hospitals in the Richmond area. When I met Carolyn she was in the process of putting together a budget for community outreach for the next year. She suggested that I write a letter explaining my proposal to prepare parish nurses for ministry in their congregations. Carolyn presented my letter to Marilyn Tavenner, who was the CEO of HCA at the time. To my amazement HCA supplied a grant of $55,000 a year for three years. The initial grant paid for my salary and the start-up resources for teaching the parish nurses. I wrote the letter in the summer of 1996 and began teaching the course on April 1, 1997! The grant was renewed in 2000 for $100,000 a year—again for three years. This money pays my salary and that of the assistant director, and pays for library resources, a newsletter, and resources to help the nurses get started within their congregations. For instance, each nurse receives a "tool box" including blood pressure equipment and a file box of health-related resources. In addition, HCA supplies scholarships to any HCA nurse who enrolls in the parish nurse program. The tuition is $800 and that includes everything—books, meals, a retreat, faculty salary, and other resources.

I am in awe about how God has worked to bring this all about. I am humbled that God has decided to use me. HCA continues to support us because the feedback is that the nurses who complete our program are changed when they return to the hospital. They form a sisterhood of support that changes the hospital units to which they are assigned. They return to their full-time jobs with a different spirit, having fallen in love with nursing again.

I coordinate the thirteen-week program that awards fifty-seven continuing education credits through the Union Theological Seminary and Presbyterian School of Christian Education. The thirteen weeks have a strong biblical and theological basis with an emphasis on God's role throughout. The participants come together one night a week from 5:30 to 9:30 P.M. During the first few weeks, they begin every meeting with worship conducted by various faculty, guest pastors, and practicing parish nurses. Then, I teach a class on worship leadership for parish nurses where I present a model of worship that suggests a pattern that is then incorporated into everything else that is taught in the remaining weeks. Once this content has been taught the nurses take responsibility for conducting the weekly class worship.

The model shows that worship is the center for healing; it is where healing begins. The model includes four elements—gathering together, hearing the word, sharing the word, and sending forth. These four elements should be present in everything that the parish nurse does, whether it is a nursing home visitation or an educational program.

After worship, the nurses share a meal together where they are frequently joined by seminary students and faculty. The meals are planned to foster spiritual reflection and growth. Every week the students are given a spiritual reflection question that they are invited to pray and think about during the week. Some nurses choose to share their reflections in unique ways—some write their thoughts in prose, others in poetry, and one student created a quilt to express her thoughts. The next week this question is put on the dinner table and students are encouraged to share their reflections from the previous week. This process encourages an intimacy and connection that is not commonly experienced. By the end of the thirteen weeks the students have formed a bond that keeps them spiritually linked long after the program is completed.

After the shared meal, class begins at 6:30 and lasts until 9:30 P.M. The classes are taught by a variety of faculty—some from the seminary, others from the Richmond community. The classes include the following topics:

- transition into ministry;
- discerning the call to ministry;
- history and models of parish nurse ministry;
- worship and healing;
- ethics from a Christian perspective;
- the mind/body/spirit connection;
- theology of health and illness;
- "Tending the Spirit" (a weekend retreat);
- parish nurse as health counselor: the ministry of presence;
- parish nurse as advocate: the ministry of justice and peace;
- parish nurse as resource: the ministry of stewardship;
- parish nurse as educator: the ministry of teaching;
- parish nurse as supporter and facilitator: the ministry of caring;
- working in a congregation: the pastoral team;
- documentation, accountability, and legal considerations for parish nurse ministry; and
- stages of health ministry, setting up your practice, and creating a caring congregation.

The last session is devoted to a banquet and a dedication service for the nurses, their families, and congregations.

Our vision is that parish nurse education is more about transformation of the individual involved in the journey—we are interested more in formation than orientation, and we view what we do more as a process for a lifelong journey rather than a program. Since the spring of 1997 we have had eighty-three graduates complete this program. They represent fifteen different denominations—but regardless of whether the nurse comes from a fundamental or a liberal theological background, the spirit of God dominates the groups. It never ceases to amaze me that when parish nurses get together it is the way the church is supposed to be, with a focus on the Lord and what we share in common rather than on the issues that could divide us. (See Appendix A for Caring Congregations: Foundations for Parish Nurse Ministry course objectives.)

God certainly does prepare those that He calls. He scatters seeds and brings forth a harvest that is beyond our imaginings. He has ordained parish nursing as a ministry and He will continue to orchestrate its development and spread it throughout the world. The varieties that exist in parish nurse preparation are a true reflection of the richness and diversity that exists within the nursing profession, within the church, and within our world. The journey may indeed lead to the same destination, but there may be many alternate routes for the trip.

CHAPTER 6

Foundation and Models of
Parish Nursing

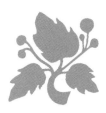

Therefore everyone who hears these words of mine and puts them into practice is like a wise man who built his house on a rock. The rain came down, the streams rose, and the winds blew and beat against the house; yet it did not fall, because it had its foundation on the rock. But everyone who hears these words of mine and does not put them into practice is like a foolish man who built his house on sand. The rain came down, the streams rose, and the winds blew and beat against the house, and it fell with a great crash. (Matthew 7:24–27)

Any homebuilder knows the importance of starting with a good foundation or base. In fact, a firm footing is necessary not only for building structures, but also for building character, knowledge, and skills. The foundation has to be solid and it has to be deep enough to support whatever is built or developed on top of it. Likewise, a sound foundation is essential to the practice of the individual parish nurse and for the specialty of parish nursing as well.

In addition to a firm base, blueprints or models aid in new construction. No contractor would begin work on a house or an office building without a plan to follow. The blueprint identifies the design elements and the major aspects of the structure and illustrates how these elements relate to one another and fit together. A nursing model is very similar in that it identifies and defines major concepts and illustrates how the concepts work together to produce a coherent whole.

When parish nursing first began with the vision of the Reverend Granger Westberg, it was well rooted within the Christian theology of health, healing, and wholeness. Westberg believed in the concept of *shalom,* meaning that a person's health was much more than physical well-being or the absence of illness. Westberg viewed the individual as an integrated whole, created to live in harmony with God, self, others, and the environment. This concept of wholeness involves freedom from physical ailments but so much more. It involves reconciliation with God, being able to give and receive forgiveness, loving and being loved, believing that one's life has purpose and meaning, and experiencing a sense of joy and hope.[1] This is a concept of health and wholeness that goes beyond what medicine alone can offer. Rather, this concept of health and wholeness is what Westberg believed the parish nurse could facilitate by linking the secular world of high technology and medical interventions with the sacred world of God, prayer, church, and community. These beliefs regarding health and wholeness and the role of the parish nurse formed the foundation upon which the first parish nurses practiced. This model, based on a groundwork of Christian beliefs, was linked to an organizational structure willing to support and extend the model.

The concept of the parish nurse was initiated as a result of a partnership between six churches in the Chicago area and Lutheran General Hospital. As noted in chapter 5, the hospital supported the original six parish nurses by paying 75 percent of each nurse's half-time salary; each church supplied the remaining 25 percent. With each successive year the hospital decreased its financial support by 25 percent while the churches increased their financial commitment by 25 percent, so that by the fourth year the churches were fully supporting the salaries of the parish nurses. As Lutheran General decreased its financial support to the original six churches, that money was freed to be used to initiate parish nurse positions in other congregations. The partnership between the churches and Lutheran General extended beyond just financial support. Lutheran General also provided resources for the ongoing development and continuing education of the nurses with half-day weekly supervision sessions held at the hospital. Westberg provided the supervision along with the hospital chaplains, a nurse from the hospital teaching program, and a doctor in family medicine.[2]

Granger Westberg described a model of parish nursing that referred to the parish nurse as a "minister of health." This model had four major functions: 1) health educator; 2) personal health counselor; 3) trainer of volunteers; and 4) organizer of support groups.[3]

As the idea of parish nursing took hold across the country, initially it remained rooted in a Christian theology of wholeness and used the model described by Westberg. However, over time the organizational structure began to change. Not every parish nurse started her ministry work within a congregation in a salaried position; not every parish nurse received the clinical support provided by Lutheran General Hospital under the guidance of Westberg. Today, almost two decades after Westberg worked with the original parish nurses, the foundation is also changing. Not every parish nurse position is based on Christian theology; parish nursing has become not just interdenominational but also interfaith in scope, with parish nurses functioning within churches, synagogues, and mosques. In fact, the term "parish nurse" is now recognized as the generic title that describes the role of a registered professional nurse working in conjunction with a faith community and operating according to the *Scope and Standards of Parish Nursing Practice*.[4]

For instance, Linda Weinberg's story provides an example of how parish nursing is adapted within a Jewish tradition. A recent article published in the *Philadelphia Inquirer* described the health ministry of Linda Weinberg.[5] Linda is one of three congregational health nurses serving Jewish communities across the country. Linda was trained in the Christian model of parish nursing at Villanova University. She then approached the Board of Rabbis about offering her services to synagogues. The only synagogue interested in her services was her own congregation of B'nai Jacob in Phoenixville, Pennsylvania. Ms. Weinberg has lined up four volunteer nurses who work in conjunction with parish nurses at a nearby Catholic parish, St. Ann's. In addition to her work with the synagogue, Ms. Weinberg is the congregational nurse for a project sponsored by the Pew Charitable Trusts. In this role she serves people of all faiths, bringing a "Jewish bent" to her ministry. She works in partnership with a Jewish community chaplain and social worker who make occasional visits. According to Weinberg, "We are packaged as a bundle with the nurse as the glue in the middle." They visit fourteen area boarding homes and minister to individuals who are damaged both physically and spiritually. Contrasted with the nurses' stories appearing in chapter 1 of this book, Weinberg describes her call in a very different manner. "I don't have the idea of a higher power who's into everyone's lives, but I do think someone's pulling the strings to make me do this. If you say, 'Do I have a Jewish calling to do this?' I say, 'Yes I do.'"

Different Models of Parish Nursing

As noted above, parish nursing today is not a homogeneous specialty. However, when asked to describe the model that they work under, most nurses who shared their stories for this book responded to that question in terms of whether they were in a paid or unpaid position. There are other features, however, that distinguish one model of practice from another.

In the early days of parish nursing, models such as the Miller Model of Parish Nursing focused on the practice of the individual nurse serving as a calling to ministry from a congregational base. As parish nursing continues to evolve in depth and sophistication, so too are the models that depict the practice. For instance, the model developed by Koenig[6] and referred to in chapter 2 illustrates the complexity of the parish nurse's pivotal role in linking the secular system of the health-care community with the sacred system of the congregation. Sybill Smith makes another distinction among different models based on the underlying philosophy. Each of these models is reviewed.

Paid versus Unpaid

Across the country the majority of parish nurses are unpaid for their church-based clinical work. This is also true of the majority of the parish nurses who responded to our questionnaire. Those that are in paid positions are generally in church-based coordinator roles over a large number of volunteers within their own congregations or in hospital-based coordinator roles over a congregational network. Linda Scott's story is a typical one.

THE MODEL I started at First Lutheran Church in Brookings, South Dakota, was a volunteer model because my congregation was struggling to stay within budget. I knew that there was no money to add expenses for a new program and a volunteer model would allow us to get started. I proposed that we operate under a volunteer model for two years, and then reevaluate. I had hoped to seek funding through a grant. Also, I hoped that the congregation would recognize the program's worth and be willing to budget at least a small portion toward materials and expenses.

My congregation of about two thousand did reimburse me for the cost of the parish nurse preparation course and for some of the supplies that we needed for our annual health fair. Also, the congregation made space and office supplies available for a little office in the "mother's cry room." This "cry room" had a restroom, a space for infants and small children, and a window to the sanctuary. It worked well as a space to conduct our Sunday morning blood pressure screening between services because it was an existing space that lent itself to multipurpose use. The other kind of support I received was encouragement from the pastors and church council for whatever health-related activities I had time to pursue.

I was the coordinator of this unpaid model. There were three or four RNs with current licenses who worked with me. In addition, I had the support of two retired RNs and two or three other women who were interested in serving as health volunteers. We operated under this model from August 1993 through May 1998. At that time, I moved away to another state. We must have gained the trust of the congregation, though, because after I left an arrangement was worked out with the hospital and a new parish nurse was hired.[7]

Rosemarie Matheus, one of the pioneers in parish nurse preparation and the director of the Parish Nurse Institute at Marquette University School of Nursing, was asked about models of parish nursing. She too responded regarding whether or not the nurse is paid.

WHEN I AM TEACHING students who are enrolled in my parish nurse preparation course, I encourage them to avoid the term "volunteer model." When people are describing a volunteer model, there is frequently a negative connotation to "just being a volunteer." I always suggest that nurses should make the distinction between paid and unpaid with the hope that if they are in an unpaid position there is always the possibility that it will become a paid position.

I definitely have a bias for the paid model. I have worked with both of these models and find that there are problems with the unpaid model, especially if a hospital is supporting it. There is nothing beyond the spirit of the individual nurse that compels the nurse to put in a certain number of hours, to maintain a documentation system, or to meet any of the hospital's quality issues. If a hospital system is supporting an unpaid parish nurse program under the umbrella of the hospital, it raises serious ethical questions.

I have heard people say that the church must make a financial contribution to the salary of the parish nurse. Although I believe the parish nurse should be paid, the salary can come from either the church, the hospital, or from both. I have observed quite a few situations where the church has paid nothing and this has not seemed to influence whether or not the congregation respected the contributions of the parish nurse or even if the role of the parish nurse was fully integrated into the ministry program of the congregation.

I suggest to my students that if their church says that it cannot "afford" a parish nurse, that they enter into a covenant with the congregation. They offer to work for nine to twelve months in a pilot role. At the end of the pilot program, the church then reevaluates the value of the parish nurse's contributions. If the church believes that the parish nurse is making important contributions, then the contract is rewritten and a salary is agreed upon. Initially, the salary may not be what the nurse might receive in the open market place but it is a start. I have found that in 90 percent of these situations, churches are willing to pay the nurse.[8]

Model Depicting Individual Parish Nurse Function

There are a number of good examples of these types of models.[9] One of the earliest was created by Dr. Lynda W. Miller as part of her doctoral dissertation and was published in the Winter 1997 issue of *Journal of Christian Nursing*.[10] The Miller Model is a general nursing theoretical framework clearly grounded in Christian faith. It provides a foundation for parish nursing practice, education, and research. Miller believes it can also serve nurses in any setting where they practice from their evangelical Christian worldview. She displays her model in the form of three stained glass windows, each depicting a different aspect of parish nursing. The first stained glass window depicts the concepts central to all nursing practice—the nurse (parish nurse), health (depicted in terms of the Christian tradi-

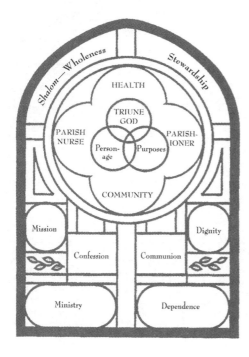

In the figure (stained glass window): Shalom—Wholeness, Stewardship, HEALTH, TRIUNE GOD, PARISH NURSE, PARISH-IONER, Person-age, Purposes, COMMUNITY, Mission, Dignity, Confession, Communion, Ministry, Dependence

FIG. 6.1.Components and major concepts of the model. *Used with permission by Lynda W. Miller, RN, Ph.D. First appeared in* Journal of Christian Nursing, *Winter 1997, 17–20. e-mail jcn@vcf.org.*

tion of *shalom*), the context of care (the community), and the person receiving care (the parishioner). In the center of the first stained glass window is the concept of the triune God—the Father, Son, and Holy Spirit. This theological concept of the triune God or the Trinity is a Christian truth, affirmed for over twenty centuries of church history, and serves as a unifying concept to Christians regardless of cultural and denominational differences.

The second stained glass window depicts the complex and interconnected dimensions of the person and how the person relates to health-promoting resources such as God, family, the faith community, friends, health care and social services, vocation, and recreation. In the third stained glass window, Miller shows the many contexts of the parish nurse role, including the Christian community, the health-

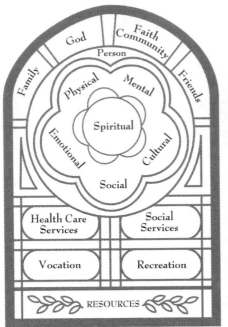

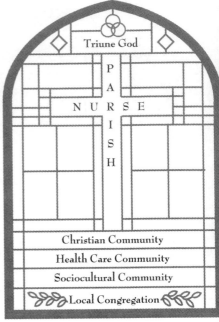

FIG. 6.2. Aspects of the whole person (spiritual, physical, mental, emotional, social, cultural) and health promoting resources of the person.

FIG. 6.3. Contexts of the parish nurse role.

Used with permission by Lynda W. Miller, RN, Ph.D. First appeared in Journal of Christian Nursing, *Winter 1997, 17–20. e-mail jcn@vcf.org.*

care community, and sociocultural communities as well as the local congregation.

Parish Nurse as Link between Sacred and Secular

A model developed by Koenig and shown in Figure 6.4 focuses on the functions of the parish nurse and clearly demonstrates the vital role that the parish nurse fulfills as the link between the church community and the health-care community.[11]

This model (also referred to in chapter 2) represents an evolu-

Functions of the Parish Nurse

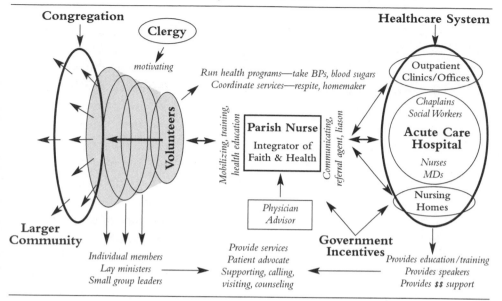

FIG. 6.4. Adapted from Koenig, H. (2001). Presented at the conference "Faith in the future: Religion, aging, and healthcare in the 21st century," Duke University, Durham, North Carolina.

tionary view of the significance of parish nursing to the health-care system as we continue to move into the twenty-first century. Dr. Koenig, one of the authors of this book, believes that parish nurses will play an increasingly critical role in the provision of health care. As the number of aged expand and their needs for comprehensive health care increase, the capacity of the health-care system to provide this care will shrink. If today's resources seem barely adequate, tomorrow's may seem scarce to nonexistent for long-term comprehensive care. The parish nurse provides an answer to this dilemma of shrinking resources in the face of expanding needs. Through the nurse's ability to train and mobilize volunteers within the church community, parish nurses are capable of providing care extenders when the traditional health-care system is stretched to the breaking point. Through her functions as educator and counselor, the parish nurse motivates and equips church volunteers to carry out preventive care activities, to provide respite for overburdened families and caregivers, to offer spiritual support, and to assist in the monitoring and management of chronic illnesses, again decreasing the burden on the traditional health-care system. This model is particularly important in congregations that contain many people with health problems needing care. If the parish nurse tried to meet all these preventive, spiritual, and health-care needs herself, she would rapidly become overwhelmed and burned out—hence the emphasis on being a trainer and motivator of volunteers. Through integrating faith and health, the parish nurse draws the power of belief, prayer, ritual, and community into the equation of health and healing.

Access, Marketplaces, and Mission/Ministry Models

The last types of models that we examine in this chapter are delineated by Sybil Smith.[12] Smith believes that as parish nursing moves more into the mainstream of health care it begins to take on a different appearance. Understanding the underlying philosophy behind various parish nursing models helps church leaders to choose a model that is congruent with their ministry goals. Smith describes three types of models: access, market, and ministry.

Access models are driven by a belief that equal access to health care is a right for all. Although access models are political in nature, they do not preclude the role of faith. However, the underpinning for the access model is not a faith-based belief in *shalom* but rather theories of advocacy, poverty, justice, and empowerment. These theories are often tied to philosophies of public health science and community health. Parish nursing becomes the mode to increase access to health care for those for whom the door to health care is often closed. The integration of faith, although possible, is not the focus of such models. In the story of Linda Weinberg presented earlier in this chapter, her work with the fourteen boarding homes in the Philadelphia area, which is supported by the Pew Charitable Trusts, is an example of an access model.

Marketplace models are tied in some way to a health-care system. In this model parish nursing is operated through home care, case management, community outreach, marketing and business development departments, and other departments within a health system. Marketplace models are driven by economic values and offer a commodity to a congregation. Sometimes the parish nurse program is used as a marketing or public relations tool with the hope of increasing the market share of the health-care system that is represented by the parish nurse. The nurse may or may not be a member of the congregation served, which means that she may or may not have a vested interest in the welfare of the community as a member as well as a committed believer. The church facility is the site for delivering health services. In-reach programs for church members as well as outreach programs to the underserved in neighboring communities are provided through the marketplace model. However, whatever is provided in some way benefits the bottom line of the health-care system. Although the term "parish nurse" is used, it is inappropriate because the nurse's main efforts are not on behalf of the congregation but rather for the health-care system. Sometimes the nurse employed by a marketplace model experiences real values conflict when indeed her motivation is ministry and her employer's is profit.

The last type of model to be discussed is the mission/ministry model. In this model the nurse can be either a paid or unpaid staff member on the ministry team of the church. The nurse who functions in a mission/ministry role has experienced "God's call" to this ministry. The focus is less on the role of the nurse and more on the persons served. Nurses feel called to be stewards of their faith and in responding to this call they find meaning and purpose. The mission of the parish nurse is to be an integrator of faith and health and in so doing to assist church members to endure the spiritual, emotional, and physical challenges of life that come to each of us. This is the model represented by most of the stories of nurses told throughout this book. These nurses join together in solidarity with their fellow parishioners, coming together in worship and prayer to share in the healing ministry of their God and their church community.

Blended Models

Many parish nursing programs represent a blend of these three models. An example of such a blended model is Mercy Hospital Parish Nurse Program, which started in January 1991. This model is primarily a mission/ministry model but it clearly has elements of the access and marketplace models as well. The program began as a community outreach with seven part-time nurses serving ten inner-city congregations in the heart of Pittsburgh, Pennsylvania. The program was undergirded by the teaching of the Roman Catholic Church and the Sisters of Mercy. Maria T. Boario was the nurse hired to be the manager of the program.[13]

> I BEGAN my second week of orientation by visiting and talking with several parish nurses and program managers in the Chicago area. This orientation, arranged by the hospital in cooperation with the National Parish Nurse Resource Center, provided valuable insights into the role of the parish nurse.
>
> When I returned to Pittsburgh, I wanted to develop a parish nurse program that reflected the uniqueness of Mercy Hospital: its long-standing commitment to the poor, its integration of mission and values throughout the health-care system and its visionary leadership in undertaking this creative outreach program. Above all, I wanted a program that would give glory to God, so I committed it to him.
>
> Next I conducted needs assessments of each parish expressing interest in the program. As I walked through the neighborhoods with the pastors, I became aware of the uniqueness of each con-

gregation, as well as the social commitment that each pastor had to his neighborhood.

For various reasons, several churches declined to participate. Some pastors felt reluctant to start a new program because of the financial instability of the parishes; others wanted to take a wait-and-see approach; another did not see the need for a parish nurse.

After careful evaluation, ten congregations were finally selected—seven Roman Catholic, two Lutheran, and one United Church of Christ—with memberships ranging from seventy-five to three thousand. Because of their geographic proximity and smaller membership, six churches would be served by three nurses. The four largest churches would each have their own parish nurse.

Selecting the parish nurses became my next challenge. In undertaking a project of this size, I believed the key to our success would be in matching the right nurse with the right church. In response to advertising in three Pittsburgh newspapers, as well as church bulletins, forty nurses applied. Surprisingly, no applicants came from the selected churches. No minorities applied either, although recruitment strategies targeted these two populations. The manager of the Pastoral Care Department and I interviewed twenty applicants and narrowed the field to fourteen finalists. The churches and their respective health committees then interviewed at least two nurses, and we mutually agreed upon the parish nurse for each church.

The hospital held a joyful and symbolic commissioning service for the parish nurses on January 11, 1991. Sister Joanne Marie anointed each of the nurse's hands with oil and the Reverend Abigail Rian Evans gave the keynote address, "Called by God." We felt a special bonding to our sisters in spirit, the Sisters of Mercy. One hundred and forty-four years after seven Sisters of Mercy founded The Mercy Hospital of Pittsburgh, seven parish nurses followed in their footsteps and tradition to provide wholistic care to the inner city.

The orientation for these parish nurses was what my colleague Jennifer Corbett, O.S.F., at Columbus Cabrini Parish Nurse Program, calls the "plunge" method. After three days of intensive inservice training, they went into the community to take the plunge. Weekly staff meetings provided peer support, collaboration/resource sharing, and spiritual formation besides sharing the successes and frustrations. Our prayer list quickly grew to include clients, friends, and families, those in authority over us, as well as ourselves.

The weekly staff meetings became a continuation of orientation and training as representatives from community agencies and Mercy Hospital came to discuss their programs and seek ways to collaborate and link resources. The resources and expertise of skilled hospital professionals greatly enhance an institutionally-based parish nurse program. Nurse clinicians, physical and occupational therapists, and pharmacists, to name a few, graciously volunteer their time and talents to assist the parish nurses with community health presentations and health fairs.

Being integrated into a health-care system means that the parish nurse may receive merit pay increases based on performance goals that are written each year. While this process continues to be refined, we have, at times, struggled to preserve the primary purpose of the program—a healing ministry—while maintaining program accountability and overall hospital corporate goals.

Program accountability also means having a system for documentation of records, monthly reports, policies and procedures, as well as a quality assurance plan in accordance with JCAHO standards. Because we are accountable to our clients, to those in authority, and ultimately accountable to God, we see these mechanisms as positive developments in achieving program excellence.

Each nurse sets her own work schedule and develops health-education programs according to the congregation's expressed needs. We make an effort to listen to the poor about what they need, following their agendas instead of ours. Four of the parish nurses provide blood pressure screenings and health-education programs at local food pantries. The only limits on this outreach are that the parish nurses do not provide hands-on nursing care nor perform any invasive procedures. The parish nurses show amazing creativity in networking and sharing what does or doesn't work for them. Two of our most common activities are advocacy and linking individuals, particularly the frail elderly, with appropriate health care and social service agencies. During the first year, providing access to health care was the most significant outcome achieved by our program.

As we look at parish nursing we see a living and growing specialty. The one constant that exists in anything that lives and grows, whether it is a person, a plant, an idea, a system, or an organization, is change. We can expect change to continue within parish nursing as it responds to various calls: the call of God, the call of the health-care system, the call of the individual nurse practitioner, and the call of the person served by this unique ministry. In the next chapter nurses describe the step-by-step process of starting a parish nurse program and the resources that helped them do so.

CHAPTER 7

Establishing a Parish Nurse Program

Steps in the Journey

 There is an old saying, "Don't go where the path leads, go where there is no path and leave a trail."[1] Many parish nurses testify to the truth of this saying as they share their stories of beginning parish nurse programs in their own congregations. The developmental process and growing pains of such a ministry are unique to each nurse and congregation. Yet there are similar steps identified by many nurses that might facilitate the passage for others.

In this chapter we examine some general steps for initiating a parish nurse program. We then turn our attention to the stories of nurses as they embarked on this journey, often without a clear path to pursue but leaving a trail behind for others to follow. Next we examine the Preston Congregational Health Program Model for Ministry, which delineates an orderly process for development, implementation, and evaluation of a health ministry. Last, we return to parish nurses themselves, who provide advice to others interested in starting on a similar path.

General Steps

The Reverend Granger Westberg identified six steps for starting a parish nurse program: 1) learn as much as possible; 2) include the pastor and other church leaders in the initial dialogue; 3) form a health committee; 4) try to establish a link with a hospital; 5) select and orient a nurse; and 6) begin the program.[2] Judy Shelly expands on these steps with the following suggestions: 1) the nurse who leads the program needs a vision for health ministry; 2) a mission statement is essential to communicate effectively the purpose and benefits of parish nursing to the governing body of the church as well as to the congregation at large; 3) initial funding must be budgeted to cover the start-up costs of supplies, education, and congregational programs; 4) personal malpractice insurance is essential for individual parish nurses; and 5) the church needs to obtain malpractice insurance, which can usually be added to the church's property insurance for a nominal amount.[3]

Under the leadership of Marianne Parker, St. Joseph's Hospital Health Center's Congregational Health Program has developed useful resources to support the steps identified by Westberg and Shelly.[4] These resources provide detailed samples and explanations of each of the steps to guide the development of a parish nurse/health ministry program. The informational packet, referred to in Figure 7.1, educates the reader about health ministry and parish nursing, the values of these programs, the history, the scope of services, and the steps to starting a health ministry/parish nurse program. The policy and forms informational guide, referred to in Figure 7.2, provides samples of documents such as mission statements and bulletin/newsletter blurbs inviting participation in health ministry.

Nurses' Stories

When we asked nurses to share their stories, we posed several questions to them: "How did you get started?" "What were your experiences convincing your parish/congregation that parish nursing was a valuable addition to the church's ministry?" "How did you introduce the concept to the church at large?" "What type of reception did you receive?"

FIG. 7.1. **St. Joseph's Hospital Health Center's Congregational Health Program Informational Packet**

1. St. Joseph's Hospital Health Center's Mission

2. Congregational Health Program Purpose

3. Taking a Look at the Public and Private Health Issues

4. Why Call upon the Faith Community?

5. St. Joseph's Hospital Health Center (SJHHC) Congregational Health Program
   a. Parish Nursing
   b. Congregational Health Ministry
   c. Education and Training
   d. Wellness Programming
   e. Agency Liaison

6. What are the qualifications to become a Parish Nurse?

7. What are the common models for parish nursing/health ministry?

8. Do Parish Nurses have to document?

9. History of Parish Nursing

10. Defining Parish Nursing: What is the role of a Parish Nurse?

11. Steps in health ministry/parish nursing program

12. Defining Congregational Health Ministry

13. How do we implement a Health Ministry/Parish Nurse Program?

14. Program Participation: SJH-HC's Congregational Health Programs Coordinator

15. Program Participation: The Local Faith Community

16. Wellness Programming

17. Agency Liaison

18. Education and Training

19. Resource Library

20. Health Fair Supplies

21. Additional Resources
    a. Policy and Forms Information Guide
    b. Health Fair Planning Guide
    c. Growth and Development Guide
    d. ANA Continuing Education Take-Home Articles
    e. SJHHC School of Nursing Library—available to parish nurses in SJHHC Congregational Health Program

22. Bibliography

Used with permission of St. Joseph's Hospital-Congregational Health; Attn: Marianne E. Parker, RN, 301 Prospect Avenue, Syracuse, NY 13203; 315-445-0915.

FIG 7.2. Policy and Forms Informational Guide, St. Joseph's Hospital
Health Center's Congregational Health Program

1. Mission Statement	7. Visitation Recommendation
2. Sample Communication with Your Congregation	8. Blood Pressure Consent/ Documentation
3. Job Description—Coordinator	9. Blood Pressure Booklet Master
4. Job Description—Parish Nurse	10. Annual Planning Outline
5. Job Description—Health Cabinet	11. Monthly Summary
	12. Annual Evaluation
6. Confidentiality Recommendation— Mandatory Reporting of Abuse	13. Health Ministry Survey

Used with permission of St. Joseph's Hospital-Congregational Health; Attn: Marianne E. Parker, RN, 301 Prospect Avenue, Syracuse, NY 13203; 315-445-0915.

Getting Started

Almost unanimously nurses told us that one of the first steps and one that they revisit throughout their journeys is the need for prayer. In addition to praying, Dr. Sagrid E. Edman suggests that nurses who are considering entering a health ministry as a parish nurse ask themselves the following questions.

- Do I have the spiritual resources to give continuously?
- Can I give up the typical nurse role of "fixer of every situation"?
- Am I a team player? Loners don't make good parish nurses nor do they facilitate a congregational health ministry.
- Am I able to be creative and think outside of the usual clinical or hospital "box"?
- Am I someone that church members will be able to trust? A congregation is not a hospital system with patients as a captive audience. Congregants will not come to something or to someone they do not trust.[5]

Another common start-up issue was preparation. The nurses who responded to our questionnaire reported that they sought out some sort of parish nurse preparation. This preparation varied from a series of one-day workshops to a semester-long course offered through a seminary or a university setting. Many attended one of the courses mentioned in chapter 5. Another frequent comment focused on whether or not the particular preparation had been endorsed by the International Parish Nurse Resource Center. Linda Scott is one such nurse who underwent parish nurse preparation.[6]

IN 1993, I took the basic parish nurse preparation class through Concordia College at Moorhead, Minnesota. The course consist-ed of four parts: 1) the parish nurse role: integrating faith and health issues; 2) wholistic health and wellness concepts for the parish nurse; 3) the parish nurse as a personal health counselor and advocate; and 4) the parish nurse working with people across the life span. Since there were so few parish nurses practicing at this time, there was no clinical component for "shadowing" a parish nurse—we just had to visualize what the role would look like. The program that I attended was later endorsed by the In-ternational Parish Nurse Resource Center but with additional classes required. I went back to Concordia to complete those classes.

Dr. Sagrid E. Edman enrolled in the course taught by Rosemarie Matheus at Marquette, also endorsed by the International Parish Nurse Resource Center.

THE COURSE at Marquette gave us almost more than we could handle, in terms of bibliographies, journal articles, health-related material, and free sources of wellness pamphlets and teaching materials. I wanted to take the course from Rosemarie. She has a very global perspective on parish nursing. I experienced a "call" to become a parish nurse while taking this course. Everything about the ministry of parish nursing fit what I felt God wanted me to do in my retirement. I didn't really learn much that was new, but the course put nursing in the perspective and context of the congregation and gave me a good feel for the roles and boundaries of parish nursing. It fit with my years as a nursing educator. It fit with what I think nursing is all about—a compassionate, caring, and healing ministry.

Convincing the Church Leadership

A successful parish nurse program and/or a congregational health ministry absolutely depends on the full support of the pastor and other church leaders. Some of the nurses reported that the idea originated with the pastor, who convinced the church leadership; other nurses needed to convince the pastor first before moving on with program development.

Judy Shelly's story is unique in that her husband, Jim Shelly, is also the pastor of her church.

OUR PASTOR (my husband) had been encouraging me to start a parish nurse program for years. Several congregational leaders had read articles about parish nursing and had begun to ask, "Why can't we do this?" So the ground was fertile. I gathered the nurses in the congregation for an informational meeting and asked for volunteers to serve on a parish nurse task force. Four agreed to serve.

Like Judy Shelly, Carole Kornelis's pastor was the impetus for her church's parish nurse program.[7]

OUR PASTOR of older adults, Pastor Eric, brought the concept of parish nursing to the ministry team. He had heard about parish nursing at a conference in the Midwest and was excited about the prospect of bringing parish nursing into our church family. He called a meeting with the nurses of the congregation and others who might be interested. He invited Carol Story, the director of Puget Sound Parish Nurse Ministries, to speak, and she showed a short video entitled "An Introduction to Health Ministry and Parish Nursing . . . The Healing Team" that portrayed what parish nursing was all about and how useful it was to congregations. The idea was accepted enthusiastically and we were off and running.

The Parish Nurse Commission of the Northwest Conference of the Evangelical Covenant Church serves Minnesota, Wisconsin, Iowa, and South Dakota parish nursing as part of its congregational health program. This group, which has been instrumental in moving parish nursing forward in these states, had an interesting start, according to Dr. Edman.

OUR DISTRICT superintendent's wife had a vision for parish nursing for several years. It began when her husband was a pastor at one of our local Minnesota churches. When he became superintendent, she began pestering him about helping churches get started with a parish nurse ministry. The way to do that, he said, was to collect a group of parish nurses, write a proposal for support and funding, and present it to the Conference Board, to which he reported. So that's what she did in the fall of 1997. She called together a group of five, all of whom had either taken the parish nurse course or were going to. Several were already in parish nurse positions in their churches. We collaborated on writing a proposal and presented it to the Conference Board, which accepted it with strong support. The proposal was for a matching grant type of funding to assist the churches to start the ministry. The funding was to support a preparation course for the parish nurse plus budget for one-time, start-up office equipment and supplies for a total of fourteen hundred dollars. Participating churches had to submit a budget showing their half of the funding.

We wrote to all the churches with information about the funding, developed a brochure, included an information sheet and articles about parish nurse ministry, and offered to meet with the appropriate committee, board, or group to explain what a parish nurse was all about. Then the task force fanned out and met with churches as we were requested. So it began, one church at a time.

All the churches were receptive, but not all could see the importance of the ministry. Those who were less supportive said things like "We go to the health club every week, so why would we need a parish nurse?" and "Everyone has his own doctor, so why would anyone go to a parish nurse to have his blood pressure taken?" Slowly, however, the concept has taken hold. Most of the pastors who have a parish nurse say that they do not know what they would do without one.

In 1997, we had five congregations in the conference that had some type of parish nurse ministry. A few were unofficial and very part time. Today we have twenty-three to twenty-five churches in the Northwest Conference with parish nurse ministries!

Introducing Parish Nursing to the Congregation

The introduction to the congregation usually takes many forms. One of the most powerful is pulpit support and involves the pastor preaching on the importance of a health ministry to the church. The pastor's support and explanation about the role of a parish nurse as part of health ministry, the importance of whole person health, and the fact that the church's mission is not just to preach and teach but to heal as well, gives immeasurable backing to a new parish nurse and a health ministry. Another approach involves inserting an announcement into the church bulletin or newsletter. A sample is presented in Figure 7.3.

We are expanding a new ministry to meet the needs of our congregation and community. This health and healing ministry will use the talents of nurses, other health professionals and lay people interested in the healing ministry of the church. We are under the supervision of deacons. We need to expand the health cabinet and reach into additional areas of church and community life. There will be an information meeting on _____ from 6–7 PM. All interested people are encouraged to attend. For more information call........

Used with permission of St. Joseph's Hospital-Congregational Health; Attn: Marianne E. Parker, RN, 301 Prospect Avenue, Syracuse, NY 13203; 315-445-0915.

Catherine Lomax spoke to her congregation during all three services. This is what she shared:

> AS I START my journey to serve you, my prayers are that we can journey together side by side. Parish nursing is an old concept brought back to meet the needs of today's churches. It involves a wholistic approach including body, mind, and spirit. We will focus on the close relationship between our faith and our health. With the support of the Health Cabinet, we will be doing a parish survey to collect information to assist us in setting up programs regarding health education and illness management, counseling, blood pressure screening, and other related health issues. I will be visiting those who are sick and shut-in to assess their health needs and to link these members with congregational and community resources. I am looking forward to meeting the volunteers of the church. As a volunteer myself, I find that volunteering provides a way of both giving to others and receiving back. I ask God to put it on your hearts to come and serve Him and to share your gifts with others in the church. I will have

office hours and my door will be open to you to discuss whatever concerns you. I am creating a brochure that I will distribute with more information about my role as parish nurse, my office hours, and telephone numbers to reach me. I look forward to getting to know and meet each of you. Thank you and God bless.[8]

The last way to obtain the congregation's "buy-in" of the parish nurse program is to talk up the ministry during informal meetings. Personally reaching out to others who have a passion for the healing ministry and inviting their participation is an effective means of increasing grass-roots support. Engaging the coordinators and members of the other ministries within the church increases collaboration and expands the scope of the services that the nurse can access. Although the list of ministries varies from congregation to congregation, the following are possible considerations for parish nurse outreach: religious education, deacons, parish or church council, Eucharistic ministers, community outreach, food pantry, social ministry, human development, Stephen ministers, life teams, caregiver committee, and lay pastoral team.

The majority of nurses who responded to our questionnaire were welcomed by their congregations. However, some, like Linda Scott, encountered a mixed response.

PRESENTING the concept of parish nursing to my congregation challenged me in ways I had not expected. I thought every nurse would believe in the philosophy of parish nursing as I did . . . that it was the kind of nursing we all longed for. But I found that my colleagues and congregational members were either all for the idea or totally against it. There seemed to be no neutral ground. Those who opposed the idea voiced concern that parish nursing would threaten the local home health agency. Others were concerned about the liability of a nurse practicing in the church. Some of the greatest advocates for parish nursing believed, as I did, that parish nurses could respond to their calling to care rather than just the need for employment.

Donna Benning describes her initial reception as one of "blank stares."

WHAT TURNED the tide for me was actually providing care for a church member and then conducting the memorial service when he died. When the congregants began to see my role in action, it made a huge difference in my acceptance within the church. Another important ingredient to my acceptance was when I started to put together small teams to assist the ill with yard work and housekeeping chores.[9]

Preston Congregational Health Ministry Model

One of the most helpful models for identifying the steps in the journey was developed by Kelly Preston.[10] The role of the parish nurse is identified as a vital component of the Preston Congregational Health Ministry Model but it is not necessarily the driving element of the model. Underlying this model is the mission statement included in Figure 7.4. This mission statement emphasizes the importance of collaboration and partnerships between faith communities and the health-care system. The model is shown in Figure 7.5.

FIG. 7.4. **Mission Statement of the Congregational Health Program**

The Congregational Health Program is committed to forming partnerships with faith communities of various denominations that are seeking to develop health ministries that promote health and healing from a whole person perspective—body, mind, and spirit.

Used with permission of Kelly Preston, RN, M.S., Congregational Health Program coordinator for the Ingalls Center of Pastoral Ministries, Baptist Health System of Alabama.

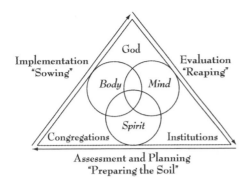

FIG. 7.5. Congregational Health Program: Model for Ministry

Used with permission of Kelly Preston, RN, M.S., Congregational Health Program coordinator for the Ingalls Center of Pastoral Ministries, Baptist Health System of Alabama.

In Preston's model, a triangle encompasses God at the apex with congregations as caring communities, and institutions such as health-care systems, universities, health departments, and other community-based providers shown at the base. In the center of the triangle is the individual church member, who is represented by the intersecting circles of body, mind, and spirit to demonstrate the individual's wholistic nature.

Outside the triangle are the steps involved in establishing a congregational ministry. Along the base of the triangle is what Kelly identifies as the first step of assessment and planning or "preparing the soil." This step is imperative and determines the success of the whole ministry. As Kelly states, "There is no point in doing surveys and programs if the congregation doesn't get it." This step takes time but it is necessary for caring, quality, sustainable ministries.

This initial phase involves a commitment from the pastor and church leadership. Not every clergyperson/pastor believes that the church has a role in health, and if this belief is absent, it is impossible to develop an effective health ministry. A health ministry team/committee must be developed with membership to include the pastor or clergy representative, health-care professionals including the parish nurse, and lay people. The health ministry team/committee provides a way to include a variety of people with diverse gifts and talents in the ministry. Training with the pastor and the health ministry team/committee is also done during this stage. Kelly identifies a number of areas where training is required: the role of the church in health; a theology of health; the relationship between faith and health; a definition of congregational health ministry and parish nursing; and the importance of assessment of needs as well as strengths, planning, and evaluation.

Included in the strategies for assessment and planning are congregational health surveys, spiritual gift surveys, data analysis of surveys, and presentation of data to the heath ministry team. (See Appendix C for the Spiritual Gifts Survey, the Congregational Interest Survey, and the Congregational Health Survey, which was developed from the Behavioral Risk Factor Surveillance Survey and includes a nine-item spiritual well-being scale.) The health ministry team then provides an overview of the data to the congregation; from this data a health ministry action plan is developed.

The implementation or "sowing" phase of the congregational health model includes the following action items: education and screenings; a course on health, values, and behavior; volunteer training with establishment of care teams; and the addition of the parish nurse to the health ministry team.

The last phase is evaluation or "reaping." Included in the evaluation phase are monthly health ministry team meetings, evaluation of all offered programs and ministry opportunities, seeking evaluation input from congregation members, follow-up surveys, follow-up screenings, and parish nurse performance appraisals.

Advice to Other Parish Nurses

Nurses shared the following advice to others interested in parish nursing.

- Pray.
- Take a parish nurse course that is recommended by its participants.

- Read everything you can on parish nursing.
- Attend at least one Westberg Symposium.
- Spend some time with a parish nurse as she "lives out" her role.
- Start small and build a foundation of acceptance.
- Build relationships—with individual church members, with existing ministries within the church, and with community resources.
- Set reasonable goals.
- Enjoy the freedom of being able to integrate your faith into your practice.
- Be strong and comfortable in your own faith.
- Be open to various forms of prayer and spirituality.
- Network with other parish nurses so you don't feel like you are "out there by yourself."
- Maintain balance in your own life—be able to say "no," lean on others, and set appropriate professional and personal boundaries.

Sometimes a journey is easy and uneventful—other times halting, slow, and uncertain. It helps to have a map; it is reassuring to know the terrain. It helps to know that someone has successfully completed this same journey before you. It helps to know that God travels with you.

Parish nurses share the map with each other. They prepare each other for the terrain. Many are far along on the journey and they beckon others to join them. All of them know that God goes before and with them.

In the next chapter we look forward to possibilities as the journey of parish nursing continues.

CHAPTER 8

Looking to the Future

The Next Generation of Parish Nursing

 It is always fun to look forward and plan for what lies ahead. We spend a lot of time musing about what we will do tomorrow, next week, next year, and even five years from now—believing we can control our destiny. Too often we are painfully confronted with the reality that our sense of control is at best illusionary. This, however, does not stop us from forecasting, predicting, and certainly not from dreaming. And so, we conclude this book about the stories of parish nurses with a glimpse into what might be, not only for individual parish nurses, but also for this new nursing specialty and for the health-care system that stands to benefit greatly from the contributions of parish nurses.

This chapter examines what we believe the future journey of parish nursing holds in the areas of clinical practice, education, and research.

Clinical Practice

In April 1997, the American Nurses Association recognized parish nursing as a specialty practice and in February 1998, it acknowledged *The Scope and Standards of Parish Nursing Practice*.[1] The Health Ministries Association (HMA) is currently investigating the possibility of credentialing as an option for parish nurses.[2] Today, as we have heard throughout this book, parish nurses are involved in improving the health of their church communities through a variety of means:

- assessing the health of the church community through blood pressure and other health-related screenings and surveys of health needs and interests;
- referring church members to community-based resources;
- acting as a liaison between parishioners and the traditional health-care system of community and hospital-based providers;
- educating about health maintenance, illness prevention, and illness management;
- advocating for the needs of congregants who lack the "medical language and/or understanding" to speak for themselves in an increasingly complex and impersonal health-care system;
- communicating health-care issues to the leadership of the church so that appropriate programs can be planned; developed, and implemented to realize fully the church's role as a healing community;
- linking the church and the health-care system—thus increasing the church's access to the expertise of those whose practices are beyond the walls of the church;
- training and mobilizing volunteers to care for one another within the congregation, to provide respite for overwhelmed family caregivers, and to fill in the gaps for long-term care that the health-care system is unable to provide;
- increasing access to health care through their outreach efforts to impoverished churches and to inner city clinics;
- counseling regarding lifestyle issues, and emotional and spiritual crises that impact on health; and
- integrating faith and health through the nurse's ministry of presence, word, and action.

These roles define the independent practice of parish nursing and exclude the dependent functions of nursing practice, that is, those functions that require a physician's order such as insertion of a Foley catheter or the administration of an intramuscular injection. Judy Shelly asserts that in the future these roles may need to expand or a different model of church-based ministry may be necessary.[3] Shelly challenges parish nurses to consider that historically the focus of nursing has been to provide care to the poor, the sick, and the disenfranchised of society—many of whom are beyond the boundaries of our churches. A nursing role that excludes nursing's dependent functions may indeed be inadequate. Shelly suggests that in addition to the independent roles of the parish nurse, parish nurses of the future may need to become more involved with physical assessment and the provision of physical care. Shelly's position is particularly persuasive in light of the predictions of the gross inadequacy of the formal health-care system to provide necessary care as we move forward.

However, rather than providing this physical care, we predict that the parish nurse will be training others to provide that physical care. Given the shortage of nurses, it will be impossible for the parish nurse to provide physical care to all the sick and old people in a congregation—there simply will be too many of them. Today the ratio of "caregiver to cared for" is five-to-one in developed countries around the world such as the United States; that figure will drop to two-to-one by 2050. There will be as many as 100 million persons aged sixty-five or over at that time—and enormous health needs in the community. The real escalation of this problem won't begin until 2011. The need for physical care will be huge.

We need members of the congregation to provide this physical care under the supervision of the parish nurse—otherwise the parish nurse will be exhausted and, like many nurses today in hospitals, overwhelmed by the physical tasks of monitoring the turning and cleaning of patients, giving nursing treatments, administering medications, checking IVs, and so on, and so on. Most of the physical care that old and sick people need is not highly skilled care, but rather simply having basic physical needs met along with caring, presence, support, and listening that anyone—especially those motivated by love of God—ought to be able to learn. Parish nurses will need to become experts in training, education, and motivation of others to carry out these tasks.

Recognition by the American Nurses Association, the existence of a professional membership organization, a formal document detailing the scope and standards of practice, plans to recognize the expertise of parish nurses through credentials, and even debate about expanding the role of the parish nurse are all signs that this specialty has achieved professional status and accountability. These achievements, so valued by the secular health-care system, are not necessarily the measure of quality within the sacred system of the church. Sometimes what the secular system promotes is clearly at odds with the values of ministry, service, compassion, love of God and neighbor, and the importance of community—all upheld by the church. Today there are nurses who are quietly expressing fears about this movement toward standardization, credentialing, and third-party reimbursement. Their voices express concern that parish nursing could become so secularized as to be no different from the disillusioning but prevailing model of nursing that currently exists in the health-care system. Their voices express a belief that the specialty is first and foremost a response to God's call and as such is primarily accountable to God and God's church.[4]

These contrasting views produce tension within the parish nurse movement.

Currently the tension is felt as a gentle undercurrent; over time the tension may pull at the fabric of parish nursing. Already there are parish nurses who are employed by hospital systems who are struggling to straddle the divide that may exist between the values and priorities of the sacred church system and the secular health-care system. This tension will only be addressed effectively if it is openly confronted with continuing dialogue between the church and the health-care system.

A current example of such dialogue exists between the Ingalls Center of Pastoral Ministries of the Baptist Health System in Alabama and various denominations within the community. The Ingalls Center of Pastoral Ministries offers a congregational health program to assist faith communities to develop whole person health ministries. Outreach is initiated to congregations by the faith-based Baptist Health System. Because both the health-care system and the church operate from a base of faith, there is a greater likelihood, although not an absolute guarantee, that values and priorities will be similar. In situations where the health-care system operates from a secular base, there is even greater need for open dialogue about the mission, philosophy, and foundational values undergirding partnerships with churches. However, we predict that the challenges of creating open communication and the potential conflict over values and mission will not impede the expansion of parish nursing and health ministries. The intrinsic value of these services both to the church community as well as to the health-care system will override any challenges that arise from these partnerships.

We also predict that as the secular health-care system recognizes the value of the parish nurse to increase the market share and the profitability of the system, there will be sharper delineation within the practice arena between parish nursing as a ministry with allegiance to God and congregation and parish nursing as a department of a health-care system. We also predict that in response to this delineation both Christian and non-Christian faith traditions will increase their involvement and ownership in parish nursing as part of wholistic health ministries, thus assuring their "place at the table" in dialogues with health-care systems regarding values and mission.

Most parish nurses practicing today serve in unpaid positions—giving freely of their time because of the strength of their call and commitment to this ministry. We believe that this needs to change and indeed will change. Parish nurses need to be paid. Whether the nurse's salary comes from the church, the health-care system, or from a partnership between the church and health-care system is not nearly as important as the fact that the nurse is paid. We tend to value things and services that cost us something, and when something is free, we tend to dismiss it as less valuable. A salary is a concrete sign that the parish nurse's services are not only important and appreciated but that the parish nurse's role is a credible and respected one within the church. Again, as churches and health-care systems recognize the contributions made by parish nurses, there will be greater willingness to budget for salaries.

Years ago the Reverend Granger Westberg wished for a thousand churches each with a parish nurse program. His wish came true. We are so convinced of the importance of parish nurses that we dare to dream even bigger than Westberg did. We dream of a time when there will be a paid parish nurse for every congregation!

Education

Many parish nurses who shared their stories reported taking a preparation course that had been endorsed by the International Parish Nurse Resource Center (IPNRC) and offered at an institution approved by the same group. The pioneering efforts of the IPNRC are to be applauded. This organization created a solid foundation for the development of parish nursing as a specialty. The IPNRC's emphasis on standardization has served parish nursing well in launching and expanding the specialty as well as in garnering professional recognition. However, there are signs that the educational preparation of parish nurses will also change as the specialty moves forward.

We predict that the changes will fall into the following four categories. First, there will be greater curricular development related to parish nursing within university-based schools of nursing with the faculty of these schools taking ownership of the objectives, content, and flow of the courses based on the scope and standards of practice. This change is in line with the traditional role of the faculty to take responsibility for curricular development. There will be clinical experiences designed for the undergraduate as well as the graduate student in nursing. At the undergraduate level, for instance, nursing students might enroll in a clinical elective under the supervision of a parish nurse.

Second, there will be an increasing number of graduate programs in parish nursing with emphasis on research into the efficacy of the parish nurse role and with recognition that the advanced practice nurse has a place within a congregational health ministry.[5] Third, there will be increased participation in the preparation of parish nurses by seminaries. An example of such participation is the course offered by the Reverend Donna Coffman at Union Theological Seminary and Presbyterian School of Christian Education in Richmond, Virginia (see chapter 5). This preparation will focus more on the theological grounding of the nurse and less on secular role definition.

Fourth, there will be more programs that meld the advanced practice of nursing with a strong theological underpinning and represent a partnership between a university school of nursing and a seminary. The Health and Nursing Ministries Program offered at Duke University and cosponsored by Duke's School of Nursing and Duke's Divinity School is one such example. This program offers three options: the first leads to a master's in church ministries and nursing ministries; the second leads to a master of science in nursing/health and nursing ministries; and the third leads to a joint master's in church ministries/master of science in nursing. Duke also offers a program leading to a post–master's certificate in health and nursing ministries.[6]

Research

A review of nursing literature reveals a growing body of research concerning parish nursing. The research points to the "youth" of the movement in that the primary focus of research efforts is on "what exists" within the field. For instance, there are studies that examine the meaning and experience of parish nursing,[7] a comparison of the roles of the rural versus the urban parish nurse,[8] an exploration of congregants' perceptions of the distinctive aspects of nursing practice within a congregation,[9] and descriptions of parish nursing practice using the Nursing Minimum Data Set.[10] However, there are no reported studies that examine the effectiveness of a particular intervention or a comparison of interventions used by parish nurses. For instance, education is reported to be an important role of the parish nurse. Does health education make a difference beyond anecdotal reports? Do congregants make behavior changes based on what the nurse has taught? Health-related screenings such as blood pressure and cholesterol levels are also reported as important interventions for parish nurses. Do these parish nurse activities lead to lifestyle changes among congregants?

Another area for research is the relationship between faith and health. For instance, a common theme among the nurses who shared their stories with us was the effectiveness of prayer and the importance of visitation to congregants either in the hospital, in a nursing home, or in the congregant's own home. An appropriate demonstration project for parish nursing might be first to examine the effectiveness of prayer. Does prayer correlate with decreased anxiety or depression? Increased hope? Increased acceptance of death? Another study might compare the effect of visitation with and without the presence of prayer. The role of the parish nurse offers countless opportunities to study the relationship between faith and various aspects of health as well as to examine the effectiveness of specific faith-based interventions such as prayer, worship service, and receiving communion. The territory is fertile with research opportunities and parish nurses have only just begun.

As we conclude this book about the stories of parish nurses and parish nursing, we hope that you have enjoyed accompanying us on this journey. The story of parish nursing is a story of call, response, journey, and faith. We began by listening to nurses describe their call to ministry. Sometimes the call was strong and clear; at other times it was vague but persistent. Likewise, the response was sometimes immediate and wholehearted; at other times it was delayed and initially tentative. All responses were acts of faith.

We listened as the nurses described the details of the journey—the highs and lows, the joys and sorrows. We heard them describe how God has led them not just to ministry within their own congregations but to ministry beyond the church to surrounding communities of need. We listened as they talked about their preparation for the journey.

One theme consistently present throughout the stories of parish nurses is that this is a ministry ordained by God. An acceptance of this as truth leads us to believe that God will continue to guide and shape this clinical practice. How it will occur is something about which we can only speculate. There is an old saying, "Man plans and God smiles." And so as we conclude this book with our predictions as well as our hopes for parish nurses and parish nursing, we can take comfort in the belief that Someone indeed may be smiling.

Parish Nursing Curricula

Concepts and Practice of Parish Nursing and Health Ministries, by Dr. Norma Small

35 Contact Hours of Continuing Education

Instructor: Norma R. Small, C.R.N.P., Ph.D. / Health Ministries Association (HMA) Consultant for *Scope and Standards of Parish Nursing Practice* / Concerned Care Management and Consultation, Inc. / 1077 Crest Avenue / Johnstown, PA 15902 / Phone and Fax: 814-539-2273 / e-mail: nrsmall@aol.com. Used with permission.

Course Description: The Concepts and Practice of Parish Nursing provides the knowledge and skills to competently practice the unique scope and standards of practice of parish nursing as described in the *Scope and Standards of Parish Nursing Practice* (HMA, 1998), and acknowledged by the American Nurses Association. Concepts from nursing, theology, medical science, psychology and sociology are applied to the unique scope of parish nursing practice. The Standards of Care: assessment, diagnosis, outcome identification planning, implementation, and evaluation are applied to the three client levels, faith community, family and individual. Emphasis is placed on integrating advanced nursing knowledge, theological beliefs and practices, and concepts from other disciplines to the implementation roles of 1) health assessor, 2) health educator, 3) health promoter, 4) health counselor, 5) teacher of volunteers, and 6) advocate. The Standards of Professional Performance: quality of care, performance appraisal, education, collegiality, ethics, collaboration, research, and resource utilization are applied to the unique specialty of parish nursing.

Objectives: At the completion of this course, students will be able to:

1. Discuss the evolution of parish nursing within the context of the history of nursing and health care.

2. Integrate advanced nursing knowledge with concepts from theology, medical science, psychology, and sociology to practice of parish nursing in a specific faith community of the student's choice.

3. Integrate the concept of health as wholeness into nursing practice.

4. Apply knowledge of spirituality, culture, race, and development stage diversity to the practice of parish nursing.

5. Implement a self-development plan in preparation as a parish nurse.

6. Use the Standards of Parish Nursing Practice: Standards of Care and Standards of Professional Performance as a tool for developing, implementing, and evaluating practice.

7. Apply the Standards of Care to the client systems of faith community, family, and individual.

8. Assess the health of individuals, families, and a faith community.

9. Demonstrate knowledge and skills as a health educator for a specific population.

10. Design a health promotion program for a faith community.

11. Demonstrate health counseling skills with an individual or family.

12. Design an education program for volunteers to meet a specific need.

13. Apply the role of health advocate to a particular situation.

14. Discuss the application of the professional performance standards: quality of care, performance appraisal, education, ethics, research, and resource utilization in the evaluation and improvement of parish nursing practice.

15. Identify the areas where the performance standards of collegiality and collaboration are important to accomplishing the desired health outcomes.

16. Discuss the advanced parish nursing practice issues: legal, professional, and ethical.

17. Discuss the role of faith communities in the changing health-care environment with the implications for parish nursing.

18. Develop a proposal to begin a parish nursing practice/health ministry program.

Content Outline:
I. Concepts of parish nursing practice
    A Parish nursing as a concept
    B. Client systems—faith community, family, individual
        1. Structures
        2. Functions

3. Interaction

4. Developmental stages

C. Communication

D. Health promotion

E. Health

   1. Wholeness

   2. Health-illness continuum

F. Health ministries

G. Caring

   1. Self-care

   2. Empowerment

   3. Mutuality

H. Spiritual development

   1. Spirituality

   2. Religiosity

   3. God

   4. Sin and repentance

   5. Forgiveness and reconciliation

   6. Faith beliefs and practices

      a) Prayer

      b) Healing

      c) Dietary

II. The practice of parish nursing

A. Standards of care

   1. Assessment—whole client system

      a) Individual—functional assessment

      b) Family systems

      c) Faith community system

      d) Health risk appraisal

      e) Resources—accessibility, acceptability

      f) Methods and tools

   2. Diagnosis

      a) Actual, perceived, or potential threats

      b) Validation

   3. Outcome identification

      a) Client's desired health

      b) Priorities

      c) Client values

      d) Measurable goals

4. Planning—spiritual, physical, psychological, social
   a) Documentation and communication
   b) Self-care actions
   c) Other care
   d) Parish nurse interventions
   e) Contingency plans
5. Implementation
   a) Independent functions of nursing
   b) Interventions
      1) Health Educator
         a) Teaching/learning skills
         b) Creativity in education
         c) Curriculum development
      2) Health counselor
         a) Individual
         b) Group facilitation
      3) Teaching volunteer health ministers and caregivers
         a) Principles of volunteer utilization
         b) Recruitment/retention
      4) Resource and referral
         a) Family, faith community, community
         b) Public, not for profit, private
      5) Advocate
         a) Identifying vulnerable persons/populations
         b) Identifying issues
         c) Organizing appropriate responses
6. Evaluation
   a) Setting criteria
   b) Cost-benefit analysis
   c) Effectiveness
   d) Documentation
C. Standards of professional performance
   1. Quality of care
      a) Evaluation of own practice
      b) Interdisciplinary/peer evaluation of practice
      c) Program evaluation
      d) Research based
   2. Performance appraisal
      a) Statutes and regulations

        b) Professional standards

        c) Employer policies

        d) Effectiveness of actions

    3. Education

        a) Self assessment of knowledge and skills needed

        b) Plan for professional development

        c) Excellence in parish nursing

    4. Ethics

        a) Ethical principles

           1) Autonomy

           2) Beneficence

           3) Justice

        b) Virtue ethics

           1) Caring

           2) Forgiveness

           3) Compassion

        c) Ethical decision making

    5. Collegiality

        a) Team work

        b) Learning from other disciplines

        c) Teaching nurses and others

    6. Collaboration

        a) Use of community resources

        b) Sharing resources with the community

        c) Working together to create needed resources

    7. Research

        a) Utilization

        b) Participation

        c) Conducting

    8. Resource Utilization

        a) Management of scarce resources

        b) Evaluation of effectiveness

III. Advanced parish nurse practice issues

    A. Legal

    B. Health-care system, current and future

IV. Beginning a parish nurse practice

    A. Proposal

        1. Purpose/goals—what

        2. Justification—why

3. Objectives—when
4. Methods—how
5. Resources needed
6. Budget
7. Evaluation plan—outcome
B. Marketing
C. Congregational ownership
V. Parish nursing future
A. Congregations as a part of the health-care system
B. Professionalism in parish nursing

Methodology: A variety of teaching methods are employed including lecture/discussion, personal logs, written papers, videos, and role playing.

Textbook: Health Ministries Association (HMA) (1998). *The scope and standards of parish nursing practice.* Washington, DC: American Nurses Association.

Caring Congregations: Foundations for Parish Nurse Ministry Course Objectives, by the Reverend Donna Coffman

Caring Congregations / Union-PSCE / 3401 Brook Road / Richmond, VA 23227 / 804-254-8070 / e-mail: dcoffman@union-psce.edu. Used with permission.

Objectives: At the end of this continuing education course participants will be able to:
1. Describe a personal call to parish nurse ministry.
2. Express knowledge of wholistic health concepts for personal development and the development of the life of their congregation and its community.
3. Integrate basic concepts of faith and health to build an effective health ministry in a particular congregation.
4. Demonstrate pastoral care skills necessary for the practice of parish nurse ministry.
5. Build a network of resources and peer support for the ongoing growth and development of their ministries.
6. Reflect the values and priorities of professional parish nursing as set

forth in the American Nurses Association's *Scope and Standards of Parish Nurse Practice,* 1998.

Each Week:
1. Worship
2. Table question (reflection question from week before plus a reflection question for upcoming week)
3. Resource display (books, pamphlets, worship aids)
4. A gift of encouragement
5. During the week, a note of encouragement

WEEK 1

Session Title: Introduction to Parish Nurse Ministry
Session Description/Rationale: This session provides an overview of parish nursing and the course to start the participant on the journey toward building a successful parish nurse ministry.
Session Title: Telling Our Stories
Session Description/Rationale: "I believe that Story is a pattern and it gives coherence to our lives." "Story is a grid . . . a divine scaffolding that organizes experience into meaningful form" (Deena Metzger in *Stories of the Spirit, Stories of the Heart*). Telling our Stories builds community. It helps us find our place in the world and meaning in our experiences. This session will explore ways that parish nurses can use stories to promote wellness.
Session Title: Discerning Your Call
Session Description/Rationale: This session invites participants to explore their sense of call to parish nurse ministry.

WEEK 2

Session Title: Who Am I?
Session Description/Rationale: Theologian John Calvin said, "In order to know ourselves, we must know God. In order to know God, we must know ourselves." The Myers-Briggs Type Indicator is one way of getting to know ourselves. Understanding how we view the world (both inner and outer world) and work with other types is critical for ministry. The MBTI may also give us a clue to the spiritual disciplines that we are most comfortable with and point out our growing edges.
Session Title: History and Models of Parish Nursing
Session Description/Rationale: This session examines the historical development of parish nursing from its roots in diaconal ministries in the early Christian church through the deaconess movement in Western Europe to

the modern practice of parish nursing in the United States, especially Virginia. Current models of ministry are explored.

Session Title: Sowing Seeds of Wellness: Worship Leadership for Parish Nurses

Session Description/Rationale: Healing begins in worship. This session offers parish nurses resources for and experience in preparing and leading worship for individuals or small groups as a way of providing spiritual care.

WEEK 3

Session Title: The Mind, Body, Spirit Connection

Session Description/Rationale: The spirit is the center of healing and wholeness. The Holy Spirit is our greatest resource for healing. This session will introduce the connections between physical and emotional health, attitude, and our spiritual lives as related to health. Community resources for addressing wholistic care will be identified

Session Title: The Theology of Health

Session Description/Rationale: Individuals interpret or give meaning to their lives out of their own experiences and belief structure. This session will help participants to understand and interpret their own attitudes and beliefs about health and illness so that they can better walk with others in the search for meaning in a time of transition or crisis.

WEEK 4

Session Title: The Faith Community's Role in Health and Healing

Session Description/Rationale: This session creates a framework using several faith traditions' views of health, healing, and wholeness. With the aid of this framework, participants can combine their own definitions of health, healing, and wholeness with their particular denomination's statements on health and wholeness and with Scripture to build a foundation for their parish nurse ministry. Barriers found in faith communities to establishing health ministries will also be discussed.

Session Title: Assessing the Faith Community: Making the Wellness Committee a Reality

Session Description/Rationale: Building upon knowledge and practice from prior nursing education and experiences, this session will allow the parish nurse to identify similarities between the assessment of a faith community and the community at large, while using the nursing process. Suggestions for the establishment of a Wellness Committee, possible roles and their importance to Health Ministry will be discussed.

Session Title: Approaches to Prayer I, II, III, IV, V

Session Description/Rationale: Using the framework described in the session "Worship Leadership for PN," participants will have opportunity to reflect on and express prayers that may be used in personal spiritual practice as well as ways to offer spiritual care to members of the congregation.

Session Title: Making Space for the Spirit

Session Description/Rationale: Through storytelling, music, reflection on Scripture and a variety of experiences, participants will explore emerging personal images that help them further explore what tends to till their spirits and what drains or takes energy from their spirits.

Session Title: Tending the Spirit: Silence

Session Description/Rationale: By engaging in an extended period of silence, participants are invited to reflect on "Prayer as availability to God," "What must I let go of in order to be available to God?" and "What do I need in order to be more available to God?"

Session Title: Theological Reflection: Spiritual/Volunteer Supporter

Session Description/Rationale: Our culture tends not to value or encourage reflection. We are more comfortable with action. As Henri Nouwen, noted Catholic author, states in his book, *Out of Solitude,* "Somewhere we know that without silence words lose their meaning . . . without listening speaking no longer heals . . . without distance closeness cannot cure . . . without a lonely place our actions quickly become empty gestures." To remain in this ministry we must continue to deepen our awareness of God's presence within it. We must recognize that "in giving we receive" not just by feeling good about it, but because we are changed in the process. This session is an introduction to a process that will help us notice and respond to God's presence in our day-to-day lives and in our ministries and methods of sharing reflections on our spiritual journey.

Session Title: Tending the Spirit: Offering Care, Receiving Care

Session Description/Rationale: Parish nurses and others who offer care often experience "compassion fatigue" or burnout. This session will explore a spirituality of care for those who seek to live out Christ's injunction to "love your neighbor as yourself" (Matthew 22:28–29).

Session Title: Tending the Spirit with Laughter

Session Description/Rationale: To explore the healing potential of laughter and humor.

WEEK 5

Session Title: Working within the Faith Community

Session Description/Rationale: This session gives an overview of systems theory and its impact on designing a successful health ministry within a particular congregation. Different approaches to understanding congregations are explored. Participants will apply concepts to their own congregations in an effort to understand how best to approach beginning a new ministry. Participants need to have basic data about their congregation on hand for this session.

WEEK 6

Session Title: The Role of the Parish Nurse: Counselor: The Ministry of Presence

Session Description/Rationale: A major function of the parish nurse is to act as health counselor and consultant, assisting members of the congregation to express feelings, walking with them through their wilderness times, and empowering them to problem solve. The parish nurse refers members to appropriate mental health services as needed. A parish nurse is not a licensed mental health counselor or psychotherapist. However, the parish nurse must be able to communicate in a compassionate, direct, helpful way in order to facilitate wholistic health in the congregation. The parish nurse often comes to the ministry from a task-oriented work situation. This session provides a model for helping participants move from "doing for" others to "being with" others. *Listening and Caring Skills in Ministry* by John Savage is the text for these sessions.

WEEK 7

Session Title: The Role of the Parish Nurse: Advocate

Session Description/Rationale: In the late 1700s, Thomas Paine said, "Give to every other human being every right that you claim for yourself." Advocacy is a tool the parish nurse uses to weave together the scattered resources in a congregation and community. Advocacy can:

- Build bridges across barriers
- Ease the way for others
- Build the capacity and increase the abilities of others

An advocate sets an example for others to follow through:

- Coordination of divergent interests and resources
- Exertion of influence
- Education

This session will explore personal, cultural, and faith-based aspects of advocacy.

WEEK 8

Session Title: The Role of the Parish Nurse: Resource and Referral: Making Connections and Building Bridges

Session Description/Rationale: The most frequently asked questions of a parish nurse are: "Where can I find . . . ?" "Who can I call about . . . ?" This session provides participants with tools that will enable them to become a "Resource Detective." Knowing when, how, and where to refer a member of a congregation to appropriate health services is essential. A process for referral is suggested. Local, regional, and national referral resources are presented. Each participant will provide one resource to the class to help classmates begin a health resource library in their congregations.

WEEK 9

Session Title: Parish Nurse as Educator: Health Education and Promotion for the Congregation

Session Description/Rationale: Parish nursing truly involves health care as opposed to illness care. The church has a vital role to play in keeping people healthy as a part of wholistic ministry. In a paper presented at the Mayo Clinic in 1996, David Larson cited that studies have linked spirituality and churches to better control of hypertension, healthier behaviors in college students, lower suicide rates, diminished pain for people living with cancer, and fewer psychological disorders when encountering the stresses of illness. Parish nurses are the leaders of health promotion and maintenance in their local congregations and their communities. This session will review basic health promotion strategies. Resources for health promotion programs and materials will be presented along educational models and methods.

Session Title: Using Educational Mediums Effectively

Session Description/Rationale: The communication mediums used by parish nurses are so familiar that we overlook key elements in their educational use. In this session, we'll look at those mediums through the lens of effective teaching.

WEEK 10

Session Title: Integrating Faith and Health: Support Groups in the Church and Community

Session Description/Rationale: Knowledge of available systems of support is vital to the parish nurse. This session will acquaint participants with support groups already in existence and with the process for beginning a support group in a congregation to meet identified needs.

Session Title: Working with Volunteers in the Church

Session Description/Rationale: One of the functions of a parish nurse is to enable people to assist in health ministries with the congregation and community. This session describes the role that volunteers play in organizing a successful health ministry in a local congregation. Attention is given to recruitment, training, nurturing, and evaluating volunteers in the faith community.

WEEK II

Session Title: Ethical Decision Making in the Faith Context

Session Description/Rationale: This session will explore several models for ethical decision making, and will apply these models to the practice of parish nursing. Case studies will provide experience for participants in using these models. A values history form will elicit from participants current issues where ethical decisions are explored.

Session Title: Accountability, Documentation, and Legal Considerations for Parish Nurses

Session Description/Rationale: As in all sessions, the *Scope and Standards of Practice for Parish Nursing* guides this session. Participants will explore the concept of accountability and the relationship of documentation to the professional practice of parish nurse ministry. The function and scope of use of parish nursing documentation is discussed. Models will be presented. Legal implications are examined for the professional practice of parish nurse ministry.

WEEK 12

Session Title: Developing a Personal Philosophy of Parish Nursing

Session Description/Rationale: This session explores the importance of having a dynamic statement of philosophy to guide the parish nurse and health committee in ministry. Sample philosophies are reviewed and a process for developing a philosophy of parish nursing particular to each participant's practice setting is presented.

Session Title: Beginnings and Endings or Getting Started ("Nurses, commence your ministry!")

Session Description/Rationale: This session will review the tools to begin a faithful parish nurse ministry in a local congregation. Steps for building a solid foundation for the ministry are suggested. Writing a job description, creating an assessment tool appropriate to a specific congregation, and introducing the ministry to the congregation will be discussed. A time of spiritual reflection will provide participants an opportunity to share their spiritual journey reflections.

Partners in Parish Nursing, Inc.™

450 Ski Lane / Millersville, Maryland 21108-1995 / 410-729-5672 / 1-800-732-0285 #01 / Fax: 410-729-5674 / e-mail: Learn@Partners-ParishNursing.org. Used with permission © Partners in Parish Nursing, Inc.

What Is "Partners in Parish Nursing"?

"Partners in Parish Nursing, Inc." was founded in 1995 as a response to the expressed need of congregations. The need was for assistance in developing health ministries, guided by a capable parish nurse. Our primary response was to develop an educational program for preparing nurses to work as part of the pastoral team in a congregation.

The board and faculty of Partners in Parish Nursing began with a vision of parish nursing as a professional nursing specialty and an important lay ministry. The educational program we developed had to be faithful to both nursing and ministry. It had to meet the standards of each profession and be taught by a team of highly qualified practitioners of each profession.

SPECIALTY PRACTICE IN NURSING + LAY MINISTRY = PARISH NURSING

- Central to our work is a strong desire to begin with students who are outstanding nurses and teach them to do health *ministry*.
- We are intentionally *interfaith*, with resources and teaching methods that respect a wide variety of faith traditions.
- Our students participate in spiritual formation and learn to do case consultation using models developed by clinical pastoral education.
- Our purpose is to develop parish nurses who are *congregationally* oriented (even if the student is a hospital parish nurse coordinator). Our teaching strategy is theoretical and clinical rather than programmatic, stressing an interactive ministry to individuals, families, and communities.
- Our course is offered *only* in partnership with graduate schools of nursing and theological seminaries. Students may take the course for six academic credits or audit the course and receive 90 contact hours

of continuing education. (Maryland Nurses Association [Code Number P97-P28-901-418], which is accredited to approve continuing education in nursing by the American Nurses Credentialing Center.)

Partners in Parish Nursing Curriculum Design

1. Our curriculum design incorporates theological concepts into every lesson rather than grouping "all things religious" into one or two sessions.

2. The foundational perspective is systems theory. In each session, the topic is viewed from the vantage point of physical systems, the individual, the family, congregation, and society. For example, in the session on grief and loss we cover physical manifestations of grief, how loss is pervasive in our individual lives, the effect of loss on family relationships, caring for a congregation experiencing loss, and societal expressions of grief.

3. The congregation is the nucleus of health ministry. Congregations give birth to this ministry out of concern for the well-being of members and surrounding community. Even if the congregation finds support and encouragement from a hospital or community parish nurse coordinator, the health ministry belongs to the faith community.

4. Spiritual formation is an integral part of the student's experience. Faculty become personally involved and available as mentors, students keep reflective journals and turn them in regularly for faculty feedback, emphasis is given to practicing traditional spiritual disciplines, and each student explores his or her own faith tradition and customs.

5. The parish nursing student is learning leadership skills for developing a team effort, not learning to operate as a solo "professional."

6. Case consultation at each session invites students to experience a reflective, theological process common to clinical pastoral education. Students learn the value of peer support and feedback and the importance of theological reflection. This experience forms the basis of ongoing support for practicing parish nurses.

7. Students with a bachelor's degree are encouraged to take the course for six graduate credits. Registered nurses who have a diploma bring rich life experiences to the class and receive continuing education credits and a certificate. Credit students are required to write papers demonstrating their ability to reflect, do research in a theological library, and analyze a clinical situation as a "nurse in ministry."

8. Faculty are experienced in congregational health ministry and meet the qualifications necessary to teach a graduate school course. The teaching

team consists of at least one nurse with a master's or doctoral degree and one pastoral theologian with a doctoral degree.

Course Summary
Call and Vocation in Health Care Ministry

Students examine their own call to nursing; scriptural examples of call; the roots of nursing in the faith community; the vocation of parish nursing; and an introduction to the theological concept of salvation.

The Practice and the Practitioner of Parish Nursing

Beginning with the *Scope and Standards of Practice for Parish Nursing*, students learn how to begin and sustain health ministry in a faith community. Topics include the congregation as an environment for practice; building a supportive base; introducing the concept to the congregation; "programming" vs. ministry; models; documentation; issues of confidentiality; liability and insurance.

Theological Concepts for Health Ministry

After identifying spiritual issues that have emerged for them in clinical situations, students are introduced to basic theological concepts in the Jewish and Christian faiths (salvation, sin, illness, health, suffering, hope) and to the process of theological reflection.

Psychoneuroimmunology (Body-Mind-Soul and Health)

Students describe the concept of target organ systems and the connection between the mind, body, and spirit in relation to the autonomic, endocrine, and immune systems. Application is then made to the influence of spiritual practices on these systems and the impact of the mind-body-spirit connection in their personal life stories.

The Faith Community as a Social System

After reviewing basic systems theory, students apply it to life in a congregation. Included are an application of ten system dynamics to working with individuals, families, and congregations, and an introduction to the theological concept of "community." Students learn how to identify healthy and unhealthy congregational functioning. The impact of political and economic systems on health care is introduced along with the role of *Healthy People 2010* (published in 2001) and the role of religious denominations in this project.

The Human Side of the Congregational System

Acknowledging the presence of troublesome people in congregational practice as well as traditional health-care settings leads students into a look at their preferred style of responding to conflict. Alternative strategies and their appropriate uses are discussed. The implications of one's own strengths for functioning on a team are also considered. The "prophetic" role of a parish nurse is described as one approach to conflict within culture.

Assessment as Listening

Students apply the principles of community health assessment to a faith community. They identify physical assessment skills required for parish nursing and evaluate their own ability to use those assessment skills. Assessment is identified as a form of "listening" to the community, families, and individuals. Students demonstrate the ability to use active listening skills in health counseling.

Faith Development and Spiritual Assessment

Fowler's theory of faith development is analyzed in comparison with Erickson's stages of human development. Students are introduced to various tools for spiritual assessment and their appropriate and inappropriate uses.

Ethics and Congregational Health Ministries

Students identify ethical dilemmas in the contemporary health-care system. After an introduction to the virtue ethics and basic ethical decision-making parameters, students apply ethical decision making to a clinical health-care dilemma. This unit also includes the role of faith and hope and distinguishing between legal and ethical issues.

Effective Use of Prayer and Religious Ritual

After identifying ways in which prayer contributes to healing, students apply the practice of prayer in various settings in ways that accommodate the others' needs and values. Rituals are identified as an important element in human behavior. Extremes and inappropriate uses of religious rituals are identified, as will as helpful rituals for healing, wholeness, and life transitions. The parish nurses' responsibility to respect boundaries and value all faith traditions is affirmed.

Grief and Loss

By far, issues of loss accompany most situations presented to a parish nurse. Students learn to identify experiences of loss broadly and to understand the tasks of grief. Loss and grief are also identified in the life of congregations and community. A range of healing responses available to the parish nurse and health-care ministries are explored.

Health Promotion and Health Counseling

Real-time, personal application of health promotion principles is emphasized in contrast to the popular "generic" pamphlet/health fair model. Students apply Becker's model and the Precede-Proceed model to clinical situations commonly encountered by congregational parish nurses. The difficulty of evaluating outcomes in parish nursing and the importance of evaluating outcomes is analyzed. Theological concepts explored are those that support healthy lifestyle and interpret the difficulty of lifestyle change. Content includes an introduction to *Healthy People 2010*.

Self-Care for Parish Nurses

Students complete a personal wellness inventory and select one area in their own behavior to work on in consultation with a peer. Aspects of compassion fatigue are explored along with an examination of the dangers involved in a dual-caring career. Students complete this unit with a day set aside for "self-care."

Working with Volunteers and Community Resources

Leadership skills in parish nursing include working as a team member and recruiting, training, and supporting volunteers. Students describe elements in a successful working relationship with volunteers. The importance of developing an information bank of community resources is reviewed along with recommendations for making personal connections with helping professionals in the community. Students outline a process for evaluating community resources and demonstrate the ability to make an effective referral.

Integration and Evaluation

Students experience writing a job description and negotiating for an employed or volunteer position in parish nursing. The current state of the profession of parish nursing is reviewed and students are encouraged to make a contribution to the future of the profession through research. Evaluation of the curriculum, the course experience, the faculty takes place along with an affirmation of the gifts and "growing edge" of each student.

Resources for Parish Nursing

Associations/Organizations

American Nurses Publishing / 600 Maryland Avenue, SW, Suite 100 West / Washington, DC 20024-2571 / 800-637-0323 / www.nursingworld.org

This organization offers excellent written resources.

Australian Faith Community Nurses Association (AFCNA) / Anne van Loon RN, Ph.D., MRCNA / Director of Development, AFCNA / South Australia / Phone (08) 8278 8274 / Fax (08) 8278 8287 / Antonia, VanLoon / @flinders.edu.au

Health Ministries Association / P.O. Box 7187 / Atlanta, GA 30357-0187 / 800-280-9919

Health Ministries Association is a professional membership organization for parish nurses as well as other individuals involved in health ministry (e.g., ministers, pastoral counselors). It offers a worldwide support network for people of faith who promote whole person health through places of worship and in the communities they serve.

Health and Welfare Ministries / General Board of Global Ministries / The United Methodist Church / 475 Riverside Drive / New York, NY 10115-0122 / 212-870-3909

Health and Welfare Ministries provides resources and consultants to assist local churches, annual conferences, racial/ethnic caucuses, and other United Methodist programs.

The Interfaith Health Program / Rollins School of Public Health of Emory University / 750 Commerce Street, Suite #301 / Decatur, GA

30030 / 404-592-1461/Main Number Fax: 404-592-1462 / Contact: Gary Gundersen at 404-592-1465 / www.ihpnet.org

The Interfaith Health Program focuses on a broad range of activities challenging faith groups to explore opportunities in health, especially through collaboration.

Grant Funding

The Robert Wood Johnson Foundation sponsors a grant program called Faith in Action, which awards grants of $35,000 to interfaith coalitions that include a range of religious organizations that is broadly representative of the faith traditions within the community. Participation by other organizations such as social service agencies, civic organizations, and hospitals is also encouraged. Faith in Action is built on the values that all religions share a mandate to do good works by helping those who need assistance. The proposed coalition must plan to do the following:

• serve a geographic area with at least 20,000 people;
• recruit volunteers from all walks of life (a commitment to others is a requirement for volunteers; formal religious ties are not required);
• organize and train volunteers to provide services to homebound individuals who are frail and elderly or affected by long-term health problems as well as provide respite for those who care for a homebound family member;
• serve people of all ages and faiths who suffer from long-term health problems of all kinds, ensuring that no person is denied participation as a caregiver or a recipient of services based on age, race, religion, or sexual orientation;
• develop a system for making referrals to and receiving referrals from the formal health-care system;
• establish a board of directors or a special advisory board for the program;
• employ a full-time director who will work with religious institutions, develop relationships with community organizations, and manage recruitment, training, and other activities to support Faith in Action volunteers;
• and secure additional resources over and above the foundation's start-up funds during the program's first eighteen months of operation.

Proposed programs are evaluated on how well they are prepared to meet these expectations.

The Robert Wood Johnson Foundation will award grants of $35,000 every four months until 2006. To apply for a Faith in Action grant, contact

the National Program Office toll free at 877-324-8411 or visit www.
FIAVolunteers.org.

Health Ministry Resources: Publications and Books

1. "Congregational Health Ministries—Resource Packet." This guide for congregations is available from Health and Welfare Ministries, General Board of Global Ministries, The United Methodist Church, 807 Neck Rd., Riverton, RI 02878. 401-625-5132.

2. "Lafiva—A Whole Person Health Ministry." Available from Brethren Press, 1451 Dundee Avenue, Elgin, IL 60120. 1-800-441-3712.

3. "Project LIFE—A Congregational Wellness Ministry." Available from 6901 North 72nd Street, Omaha, NE 68122. 402-572-2596.

4. "Wellness Ministry: A Partnership Program." Available from Community Outreach Pastoral Care Department, 2351 E. 22nd Street, Cleveland, OH 44114. 216-363-3311.

5. "How to Get the Church to Support and Perpetuate New Health and Human Service Interventions." Available from the Community Development and Training Center, P.O. Box 712, Carrboro, NC 27510-0712. 919-929-4527.

6. *Deeply Woven Roots: Improving the Quality of Life in Your Community* by Gary Gunderson. Available from Augsburg Fortress Publishers, Box 1209, Minneapolis, MN 55440. 800-328-4648.

Health Resources: Educational, Patient Services

A search of the internet using search terms such as patient education, or the name of a particular diagnosis or organization yields an abundance of resources and information on obtaining additional resource/teaching materials, much of it free.

American Association of Retired Persons (AARP): 1-800-424-3410

Health advocacy services provides information on long-term care, caregiving, medical decision making, health promotion, Medicare and supplemental insurance. May request catalog of publications and AV programs. Several pamphlets are free in limited quantities.

American Cancer Society: 1-800-ACE-2345 / website: www.cancer.org

A nationwide, community-based voluntary health organization dedicated to

eliminating cancer as a major health problem by preventing cancer, saving lives, and diminishing suffering from cancer through research, education, advocacy, and service.

Eldercare Locator: 1-800-677-1116

This national toll-free number connects you to the Area Agency on Aging serving the community where the person you are caring for lives.

Parish Nurse Conferences

The Granger Westberg Symposium was held every year in September. It was sponsored by the International Parish Nurse Resource Center, which closed in mid-October 2001. As a result, the future of this important symposium is unknown.

Presbyterian Parish Nurse Network

This biannual conference is held in late June and October in Santa Fe, New Mexico, and Stony Point, New York. For additional information please contact the Reverend Donna B. Coffman at 800-254-8070 or dcoffman@union-psce.edu.

United Church of Christ Annual Parish Nurse Conference / Alvyne Rethemeyer, Parish Nurse Coordinator / Deaconess Health System Parish Nurse Program / 6150 Oakland Avenue / St. Louis, MO 63139 / 314-768-3000

Parish Nurse Preparation

There is a wealth of educational opportunities and resources available on the internet. Searching on the phrase "parish nurse" opens up a cornucopia of resources. For information regarding the basic nurse preparation courses and the coordinator courses that were endorsed by the International Parish Nurse Network/Resource Center, call the number listed under associations and organizations.

Basic Parish Nurse Preparation Courses

Basic parish nurse course modules include the following:

• The Role of the Congregation in Health, Healing, and Wholeness
• Theology of Health, Healing, and Wholeness
• History and Philosophy of Parish Nursing
• Ethics in Parish Nursing
• Self-care for Parish Nurses

- Assessment: Individual, Family, Congregation
- Accountability and Documentation
- Function of the Parish Nurse: Integrator of Faith and Health
- Function of the Parish Nurse: Personal Health Counselor
- Function of the Parish Nurse: Health Educator
- Function of the Parish Nurse: Coordinator of Volunteers
- Function of the Parish Nurse: Developer of Support Groups
- Function of the Parish Nurse: Health Advocate
- Getting Started
- Functioning within a Ministerial Team
- Health Promotion and Maintenance
- Prayer and Worship Leadership
- Legal Considerations for Parish Nurses
- Grant Writing for Parish Nurses
- Grief and Loss

The following institutions were approved by the IPNRC and utilize the curriculum endorsed by the IPNRC.

Augustana College / Department of Nursing / Parish Nursing Center / 2001 S. Summit Avenue / Sioux Falls, SD 57197 / Contact: Mary Auterman / 605-336-4929

Boston College / School of Nursing / 140 Commonwealth Avenue Chestnut Hill, MA 02467 / Contact: Susan Chase / 617-552-4250

The Deaconess Foundation / Deaconess Parish Nurse Program / 211 N. Broadway, Suite 1250 / St. Louis, MO 63102 / Contact: Alvyne Rethemeyer / 314-918-9575

Edison Community College / 8099 College Parkway, SW / Fort Myers, FL 339919 / Contact: Shirley Ruder / 941-489-9214

Inter-Church Health Ministries / 71 Simcoe Street South / Oshawa, Ontario / Canada L1H G4 / Contact: Gail Brimbecom / 905-436-1572

Marian College / 3200 Cold Spring Road / Indianapolis, IN 46222 / Contact: Carol Lee Cherry / 317-955-6130

Marian College—Appleton Center / 2701 N. Oneida / Appleton, WI 54911 / Contact: Carol Burns / 920-749-1045

Marquette University / College of Nursing, Outreach Office / P.O. Box 1881 / Milwaukee, WI 53201 / Contact: Rosemarie Matheus / 414-288-3802

Medical University of South Carolina / 99 Jonathan Lucas Street / Charleston, SC 28425 / Contact: Ann Hollerbach / 843-792-4624

National Episcopal Health Ministries / 10 West 61st St. / Indianapolis, IN 46208 / Contact: Jean Denton / 317-253-1277

Northwest Parish Nurse Ministries / 2801 N. Gantenbein, Room 1072 / Portland, OR 97227 / Contact: Annette Stixrud / 503-413-4920

Nurse Ministries Network / 555 West Glendale Avenue / Phoenix, AZ 85004-1506 / Contact: Pat Midkiff / 602-274-5022

Parish Nurse Center / Carroll College / 1601 N. Benton Ave. / Helena, MT 59624 / Contact: Dr. Cynthia Gustafson / 406-447-5494

The Parish Nursing Center / Concordia College / 901 8th Street / Moorhead, MN 56562 / Contact: Jean Bokinskie / 218-299-3893

Puget Sound Parish Nurse Ministries / 502 48th Place SE / Everett, WA 98203 / Contact: Carol Story / 425-259-5809

Samuel Merritt College / 470 Hawthorne Avenue / Lakeland, CA 94609 / Contact: Joan Bard Stone / 510-869-8620

Shenandoah University / 1775 N. Sector Court / Winchester, VA 22601 / Contact: Martha Erbach / 540-665-5505

St. Joseph's Mercy of Macomb / 42669 Garfield, Suite 323 / Clinton Twp., MI 48038 / Contact: Mary Ann Stockwell / 810-412-2108

St. Scholastica College / 1200 Kenwood Avenue / Duluth, MN 55811 / Contact: Marge Monge / 218-723-6396

University of Colorado / School of Nursing / 4200 E. 9th Avenue, Box C288 / Denver, CO 80262 / Contact: Dr. Nancy Brown / 303-325-4248

University of the Incarnate Word / 4301 Broadway / San Antonio, TX 78209 / Contact: Dr. Jean Deliganis / 210-829-3974

University of Indianapolis / School of Nursing / 1400 East Hanna Avenue / Indianapolis, IN 46227 / Contact: Cheryl Larson / 317-788-3503

Viterbo University / 815 S. 9th St. / LaCrosse, WI 54601 / Contact: Ruth Williams / 608-796-3587

Waynesburg College / Department of Nursing / Waynesburg, PA 15370 / Contact: Joy Burt Conti / 724-852-3329

West Virginia University / School of Nursing / P.O. Box 9610 / 6404 Health Sciences South / Morgantown, WV 26506 / Contact: Debra Harr / 304-293-1590

William Jewell College / 500 College Hill / Liberty, MO 64068 / Contact: Shirley Hill / 816-415-7704

Basic Parish Nurse Coordinator Preparation Courses
 The following institutions offer basic coordinator courses that were endorsed by the International Parish Nurse Resource Center.

The Parish Nursing Center / Concordia College / 901 8th Street / Moorhead, MN 56562 / Contact: Luella Vitalis / 218-299-3893

Parish Nurse Resources
Interfaith Health Program / Rollins School of Public Health / Emory University / 750 Commerce Drive / Suite 301 / Decatur, GA 30030 / 404-420-5151
 "Getting Started"
 "The Challenges of Faith and Health" (quarterly)
 Starting Point: Empowering Communities to Improve Health

National Health Ministries Association / P.O. Box 7187 / Atlanta, GA 30357 / 1-800-280-9919 or 404-607-9357 / e-mail: hmassoc@mindspring.com
 Beginning a Health Ministry Manual

Parish Nursing Church Resource Manual / Adventist Health System West 2100 Douglas Blvd. / Roseville, CA 95661 / 916-781-2000

Parish Nurse Tools
 1. Congregational Interest Survey (see p. 172).
 2. Congregational Health Survey (see p. 173).

3. Domestic violence worship service for leader and participants (see p. 186).

4. Gerontological Pastoral Care Institute Spiritual Life Review and Needs Assessment (see p. 180).

5. Spiritual Gifts Survey (see p. 183).

Videos

1. *Congregations Who Care: The Ministry of Health and Wholeness.* This video presents parish nursing as one style of congregational health ministry. Available from Office of Media Services and the Office of Health Ministries, Presbyterian Church (U.S.A.), 100 Witherspoon Street, Louisville, KY 40202-1396. 1-800-325-9133 or 502-569-8100.

2. *Life Abundant: Celebrating Health, Healing and Wholeness.* Available from the Presbyterian Church (U.S.A.). 1-800-325-9133.

3. *Your Health Care: Too Soon to Compromise.* Available from Office of Communications, United Church of Christ, 700 Prospect Avenue, Cleveland, OH. 216-736-2222, Fax: 216-736-2223.

4. *The Healing Team: An Introduction to Health Ministry and Parish Nursing.* Available from Bay Area Health Ministries, 70 West Clay Street, San Francisco, CA 94121. 415-221-3693.

Volunteer Training Resources

1. "Called to Care: A Notebook for Lay Caregivers." Available from United Church Resources, 800 North Third Street, St. Louis, MO 63102. 1-800-325-7061. This manual contains training programs and start-up helps for a lay caregiving program. It is also helpful for parish nurses to train volunteers. Cost: $49.95 plus $6.00 for shipping and handling.

2. Carter, Rosalynn (1994). *Helping Yourself Help Others: A Book for Caregivers.* Times Books: New York. Available at many bookstores. Cost: $20.00.

3. "What to Do Until Help Arrives," a program designed by the American Red Cross to prepare nonmedical people waiting for emergency personnel to arrive after dialing 911. Suitable for training ushers in order to establish an emergency response team to respond to crises occurring on the church grounds.

4. National Family Caregivers Association (1996). *The Resourceful Caregiver.* Mosby Lifeline: St. Louis. To order call 1-800-426-4545. Cost: $12.95.

Sample Surveys and Assessment Tools

Congregational Interest Survey

The Health Ministry is interested in organizing some programs that are of interest to members of the congregation and that focus on health promotion from a whole person perspective—body, mind, and spirit. You can help us plan for these programs by completing this brief survey. Please place a check by topics that you would be interested in learning more about.

__ Adolescent health issues
__ Advance directives/Living wills
__ Alcohol/drug abuse
__ Alternative and complementary therapies
__ Anxiety disorders
__ Arthritis
__ Cancer
__ Cardiopulmonary resuscitation (CPR)
__ Caring for aging parents
__ Dementia/Alzheimer's disease
__ Dental health
__ Depression
__ Diabetes
__ Eating disorders
__ Exercise and health
__ Eye diseases/vision problems
__ Forgiveness
__ Grief and loss
__ Heart disease and stroke
__ Hypertension (high blood pressure)

__ Immunizations/vaccinations
__ Managing your medications
__ Men's health issues
__ Nutrition and health
__ Osteoporosis
__ Pain management
__ Pregnancy
__ Relationship between faith and health
__ Respiratory/lung diseases
__ Sleep disorders
__ Smoking cessation
__ Stress management
__ Support group (Types?_____
_____)
__ Talking with your doctor
__Vitamins and herbal supplements
__ Weight control
__ Women's health issues
__ Other ideas _____
_____
_____

What day(s) and time(s) would be best for you to attend a class, program, workshop, or support group?

__ Monday	__ Morning
__ Tuesday	__ Afternoon
__ Wednesday	__ Evening
__ Thursday	
__ Friday	
__ Saturday	
__ Sunday	

Used with permission of Congregational Health Program, The Ingalls Center of Pastoral Ministries, Baptist Health System of Alabama.

Baptist Health System Congregational Health Survey

Used with permission of Congregational Health Program, The Ingalls Center of Pastoral Ministries, Baptist Health System of Alabama.

Dear Congregation Member:

The purpose of this survey is to help you identify your congregation's health needs so that you can more effectively minister to your congregation and community.

Your answers to this questionnaire will be kept in strictest confidence. Your answers will be combined with that of others so that individual responses cannot be identified. All responses will be presented in a summarized report.

There is no cost to the church for this study. Rather, this survey is merely an extension of the Mission of the Baptist Health System to promote health and healing in people's lives.

Please take the time to complete this survey and answer all questions to the best of your ability. If you would like more information about this study, please fell free to call the church office.

Thank you for your willingness to participate.

Please answer every question by marking or checking one circle. If you are unsure about how to answer, please give the best answer you can.

Section I: Spiritual Well-Being

Please rate your agreement or disagreement with each statement listed below.

	Strongly Agree	Somewhat Agree	Neither	Somewhat Disagree	Strongly Disagree
1. Prayer is important in my life	○	○	○	○	○
2. I believe I have spiritual well-being	○	○	○	○	○
3. I find meaning and purpose in my life	○	○	○	○	○
4. There is a close relationship between my spiritual beliefs and what I do	○	○	○	○	○
5. I am satisfied with my life					
6. God has little meaning in my life	○	○	○	○	○
7. Prayer does not help me in making decisions	○	○	○	○	○
8. I find it hard to forgive others	○	○	○	○	○
9. I accept my life situations	○	○	○	○	○

Section II: About You

10. Are you a caregiver for an elderly parent, relative or friend? ○ Yes ○ No

11. About how much do you weigh? _____Pounds

12. About how tall are you without shoes? _____Feet _____Inches

13. Are you male or female? ○ Male ○ Female

14. Your birth year: 19____

15. What do you consider the number one health problem in the community where you live?_____

_____

16. An Advance Directive is any written instruction you give relating to the provision of health care in the event you become unable to make your own decisions. Examples of Advance Directives include: Living Wills; Durable Power of Attorney for Health Care; or the Appoint-

ment of a Health-care surrogate. Do you currently have an Advance
Directive for yourself?　　　　　　　　○ *Yes*　　○ *No*

17. Your zip code: _____

Section III: Health and Daily Activities

*These next questions are about your general health. Please give the best answer
you can.*

18. In general, would you say your health is:

Excellent	*Very Good*	*Good*	*Fair*	*Poor*
○	○	○	○	○

19. The following items are about activities you might do during a
typical day. Does your health limit you in these activities? If so,
how much?

	Yes, Limited a Lot	*Yes, Limited a Little*	*No, Not Limited at All*
a. Moderate activities, such as moving a table, pushing a vacuum cleaner, or playing golf	○	○	○
b. Climbing several flights of stairs	○	○	○

20. During the past 4 weeks, have you had any problems with your work
or other regular daily activities as a result of your physical health?

	Yes	*No*
a. Accomplished less than you would like	○	○
b. Were limited in the kind of work or other activities	○	○

21. During the past 4 weeks, have you had any of the following problems
with your work or other regular daily activities as a result of any
emotional problems (such as feeling depressed or anxious)?

	Yes	*No*
a. Accomplished less than you would like	○	○
b. Didn't do work or other activities as carefully as usual	○	○

Section III: Health and Daily Activities

22. During the past 4 weeks, how much did pain interfere with your
normal work (including both work outside the home and housework)?

Not at all	*A little bit*	*Moderately*	*Quite a bit*	*Extremely*
○	○	○	○	○

SAMPLE SURVEYS AND ASSESSMENT TOOLS　175

These questions are about how you feel and how things have been with you during the past 4 weeks. For each question, please give the one answer that comes to mind closest to the way you have been feeling. How much of the time during the past 4 weeks . . .

	All of the Time	Most of the Time	A Good Bit of the Time	Some of the Time	A Little of the Time	None of the Time
23. Have you felt calm and peaceful?	○	○	○	○	○	○
24. Did you have a lot of energy?	○	○	○	○	○	○
25. Felt downhearted and blue?	○	○	○	○	○	○

26. During the past 4 weeks, how much of the time have your physical health or emotional problems interfered with your social activities (like visiting with friends, relatives, etc.)?

All of the Time	Most of the Time	Some of the Time	A Little of the Time	None of the Time
○	○	○	○	○

27. During the past 4 weeks, how often have you visited your doctor's office, the emergency room at the hospital (no overnight stay) or stayed overnight as an inpatient at the hospital for medical care?

	No Visits	1–2 Visits	3–4 Visits	5–9 Visits	10 or more Visits
Your doctor's office	○	○	○	○	○
Hospital emergency room	○	○	○	○	○
Overnight stay in the hospital	○	○	○	○	○

Section IV: Health and Daily Activities

28. Has a doctor ever told you that you had any of the following conditions?

	Yes	No
Hypertension (high blood pressure)	○	○
Heart disease like angina or heart failure	○	○
Diabetes or high blood sugar	○	○
Cancer	○	○

29. Do you now have any of the following conditions?

	Yes	No
Arthritis or rheumatism	○	○
Chronic back problems	○	○
Trouble seeing even with glasses	○	○
Lung problems, bronchitis, asthma or emphysema	○	○
Ulcers in the stomach or heartburn	○	○

30. Was there a time during the last 12 months when you needed to see a doctor, but could not because of cost? ○ *Yes* ○ *No*

31. About how long has it been since you last visited a doctor for a routine check-up?

Within Past Year	*Within Past 2 Years*	*Within Past 5 Years*	*5 or More Years Ago*	*Never*
○	○	○	○	○

32. Do you smoke cigarettes every day, some days, or not at all.
○ *Everyday* ○ *Some Days* ○ *Not At All*

33. In the past 12 months, has a doctor, nurse, or other health professional given you advice about your weight?
○ *Yes, Lose Weight* ○ *Yes, Gain Weight* ○ *Yes, Maintain Weight* ○ *No*

Section V: Prevention

	Yes, Within Past Year	Yes, Within Past 2 Years	Yes, 3 or More Years Ago	No, Never
34. Has a doctor or other health professional ever talked with you about your diet or eating habits?	○	○	○	○
35. Has a doctor or other health professional ever talked with you about physical activity?	○	○	○	○
36. Has a doctor or other health professional ever talked with you about injury prevention, such as safety belt use or smoke detectors?	○	○	○	○
37. Has a doctor or other health professional ever talked with you about alcohol use?	○	○	○	○

	Yes, Within Past Year	Yes, Within Past 2 Years	Yes, 3 or More Years Ago	No, Never
38. Has a doctor or other health professional ever talked with you about drug use?	○	○	○	○

39. About how long has it been since you had your blood pressure taken by a doctor, nurse, or other health professional?

Within 6 Months	Within Past Year	Within Past 2 Years	Within Past 2 Years	5 Years or More	Never
○	○	○	○	○	○

40. Blood cholesterol is a fatty substance found in the blood. Have you ever had your blood cholesterol checked?

Yes, Within Past Year	Yes, Within Past 2 Years	Yes, Within Past 5 Years	5 Years or More	No, Never
○	○	○	○	○

41. Have you ever been told by a doctor, nurse, or other health professional that you have high blood cholesterol?   ○ Yes   ○ No

Section VI: Prevention

42. During the past 12 months, have you had a flu shot?   ○ Yes   ○ No

43. Have you ever had a pneumonia shot?   ○ Yes   ○ No

45. How often do you use seatbelts when you drive or ride in a car?
○ Always   ○ Nearly Always   ○ Sometimes   ○ Seldom   ○ Never

46. During the past month, did you participate in any physical activities or exercise such as running, golf, swimming, gardening, or walking?
○ Yes   ○ No

47. In the past month, have you had at least one drink of any alcohol such as beer, wine or liquor?   ○ Yes   ○ No

47a. If yes, during the past month, how many days per week or per month did you drink any alcohol beverages, on the average?
Days per week? _____
Days per month? _____

47b. A drink is 1 can of beer, 1 glass of wine, 1 cocktail, or 1 shot of liquor. On the days when you drank, about how many drinks did you drink on the average? _____
Number of drinks? _____

Section VII: Women's Health

	Yes, Within Past Year	Yes, Within Past 2 Years	Yes, Within Past 3 Years	Yes, Within Past 5 Years	Yes, 5 or More Years	No, Never
48. A mammogram is an x-ray of each breast that helps detect breast cancer. Have you ever had a mammogram?	⬭	⬭	⬭	⬭	⬭	⬭
49. A clinical breast exam is when a doctor, nurse, or other health professional feels the breast for lumps. Have you ever had a clinical breast exam?	⬭	⬭	⬭	⬭	⬭	⬭
50. A Pap smear is a test for cancer of the cervix. Have you ever had a Pap smear?	⬭	⬭	⬭	⬭	⬭	⬭

51. Are you now pregnant?   ⬭ Yes   ⬭ No

51a. If yes, have you received prenatal care in the form of nutrition counseling, education or medical care for you and your baby from a doctor or other health professional?   ⬭ Yes   ⬭ No

Section VIII: Men's Health

	Yes, Within Past Year	Yes, Within Past 2 Years	Yes, Within Past 5 Years	Yes, 5 or More Years	No, Never
52. A digital rectal exam is when a doctor or other health professional inserts a finger in the rectum to check for prostate cancer and other health problems. Have you ever had this exam?	⬭	⬭	⬭	⬭	⬭
53. A prostate-specific antigen (PSA) is a blood test to check for prostate cancer. Have you ever has this blood test?	⬭	⬭	⬭	⬭	⬭

Thank you for participating in this survey!

Gerontological Pastoral Care Institute's
Spiritual Life Review and Needs Assessment

Personal Information

Name_____

Address_____

Phone_____

Initial observation: Individual is
_____ alert and oriented _____ alert and disoriented
_____ unable to communicate

Religious affiliation_____

Level of congregational activity prior to admission:
_____ active _____ inactive

Desires visits from parish clergy and/or laypersons: _____ yes _____ no

If membership is with a congregation outside the geographic area, should that congregation be notified?_____ no_____ yes

Name & Address of Congregation:_____
_____

Desire for religious participation:
_____ Attend services _____ Bible reading and/or study
_____ Chaplain visits _____ Communion _____ Confession
_____ Hymn singing _____ Prayer _____ Other (explain):

Ability to attend religious activities:
_____ needs reminders _____ can transport self _____ needs escort

Religious beliefs and perceptions:

Image of Jesus: _____ a loving, supportive friend
_____ distant, a person in Bible stories
_____ uncertain about an image of Jesus

Image of God: _____ loving, forgiving, and supportive
_____ punitive and angry _____ withdrawn, not present
_____ uncertain about an image of God

Suffering is: ____ punishment for sins ____ meaningless
         ____ an inevitable part of life that allows for growth

Salvation is: ____ assured ____ denied ____ not understood

Strength and courage received from
         ____ God ____ Jesus ____ family ____ self ____ friends ____ staff

*Favorite hymns:*_____

*Favorite Scriptures:*_____

Important spiritual experiences:
I'm going to list some activities that may relate to your spiritual life. Tell me how important they are to you now: 3 = Important; 2 = neutral; 1 = not important.
         ____ spending time thinking, meditating, or praying
         ____ enjoying beauty: art, nature, music, etc.
         ____ learning new things about your religion
         ____ attending worship services
         ____ reflecting on the meaning of your life
         ____ sharing your spiritual life with others

Are there other important spiritual experiences you'd like to tell me about?

Are there important aspects of your spiritual life that you feel you're missing now?

Spiritual life review:
1. Tell me a little about yourself and your childhood . . .
   a. How was your home heated?_____
   b. Was the center of warmth in your home? _____
   c. Who was the person of warmth in your home?_____
   d. When, if ever, did God become a person of warmth to you?
   _____

2. Tell me about your experiences in churches through your life, beginning when you were a child and on through adulthood._____
   _____

3. What were some of the most positive experiences in your life?
   _____

4. What are some of the sad experiences you've had? How did you cope with them? _____

_____

5. Who are the people important in your life now? How do they care for you? _____

_____

6. What do you think God is asking of you now? _____

_____

7. What are you asking of God now? _____

_____

Requests for the time of dying:
_____ Music _____ Clergy Present _____ Family Present
_____ Last Rites _____ Rosary _____ The Sacrament
_____ Reading of Scripture (which passages?) _____ Other (explain)

Pastoral evaluation and plans: _____

_____

Signs of spiritual strength: _____

_____

Signs of spiritual distress: _____

_____

Recommendations for pastoral care: _____

Completed by _____ *Date:* _____

Used with permission of The Center for Aging, Religion, and Spirituality, Luther Seminary, 2481 Como Avenue, St. Paul, MN 55108-1496. 651-641-1496, e-mail: Cars@luthersem.edu

Many thanks to Cheryl Hovland, parish nurse in Pelican Rapids, Minnesota, for sharing this resource with us. Cheryl can be reached at cherylhovland2@ meritcare.com.

Spiritual Gifts Survey

"Just as each of us has one body with many members, and these members do not all have the same function, so in Christ we who are many form one body, and each member belongs to all the others. We have different gifts, according to the grace given us. If a man's gift is prophesying, let him use it in proportion to his faith. If it is serving, let him serve; if it is teaching, let him teach; if it is encouraging, let him encourage; if it is contributing to the needs of others, let him give generously; if it is leadership, let him govern diligently; if it is showing mercy, let him do it cheerfully."

—*Romans 12:4–8 NIV*

Directions

Record your answer by placing the number that corresponds to the response that best describes you in the blank beside each item. Usually your first response is best. Do not skip any items. Place the score for each item in the blank on the score sheet which corresponds to the item number. Total your scores for each gift. The three highest scores indicate your primary spiritual gifts.

Your response choices are:
5—Highly characteristic of me
4—Most of the time characteristic of me
3—Often characteristic of me; about 50% of the time
2—Occasionally characteristic of me; about 25% of the time
1—Not at all characteristic of me

_____ 1. I possess a natural inclination to encourage other people.

_____ 2. I enjoy meeting other people's needs by sharing my possessions.

_____ 3. I am sensitive to the suffering of other people.

_____ 4. I take action to meet practical and physical needs instead of merely talking about meeting needs.

_____ 5. I have a strong desire for people to live holy and righteous before God.

_____ 6. I am able to organize ideas, time, resources, and people effectively.

_____ 7. I like to study and prepare for the role of teaching.

_____ 8. I have a keen awareness of the emotions of others, such as fear, loneliness, anger, and pain.

_____ 9. I have a strong desire to proclaim God's Word to others.

_____ 10. I love to examine Scripture in a logical and systematic method.

_____ 11. I experience great joy when I have the opportunity to give.

_____ 12. I can delegate important work.

_____ 13. I can identify those who need assistance in maturing their faith.

_____ 14. I like doing things for people in need.

_____ 15. I am driven to know the truth of God's Word.

_____ 16. I am successful in inspiring a group to do its work.

_____ 17. I look for ways to encourage and comfort others in my faith family.

_____ 18. I do not require prompting or recognition in order to meet the needs of others.

_____ 19. I prefer to give the maximum rather than the minimum.

_____ 20. I have insights from Scripture concerning people and events that compel me to speak out.

_____ 21. I am drawn to people who are hurting.

_____ 22. I have a strong awareness of the physical needs of other people.

_____ 23. I desire to intercede for others to be obedient to God's will.

_____ 24. I strongly believe that stewardship is based on the recognition that God owns all things.

_____ 25. I am sensitive to opportunities to help people who need comfort and counseling.

_____ 26. I love to explain Scripture in great detail.

_____ 27. I possess an unusual capacity to offer unconditional love to people.

_____ 28. I am able to make effective and efficient plans for carrying out the goals of a group.

_____ 29. I have the ability to set forth positive and precise steps of action.

_____ 30. God uses me to facilitate others to live more Christ-like lives.

_____ 31. I like doing little things that help others.

_____ 32. I have a strong desire to minister to those who are in distress.

_____ 33. God gives me boldness to declare His Word to people.

_____ 34. I desire for the body of Christ to know and understand the truth of God's Word.

_____ 35. I desire to give generously to worthy ministries.

Spiritual Gifts Score Sheet

Prophecy

5 ____   9 ____   20 ____   23 ____   33 ____   Total ____

Service

4 ____   14 ____   18 ____   22 ____   31 ____   Total ____

Teaching

7 ____   10 ____   15 ____   26 ____   34 ____   Total ____

Encouragement

1 ____   13 ____   17 ____   25 ____   30 ____   Total ____

Giving

2 ____   11 ____   19 ____   24 ____   35 ____   Total ____

Leadership

6 ____   12 ____   16 ____   28 ____   29 ____   Total ____

Mercy

3 ____   8 ____   21 ____   27 ____   32 ____   Total ____

Name:_____

Phone:_____ Birthdate:_____

My three predominate spiritual gifts are:

1. _____   Score _____

2. _____   Score _____

3. _____   Score _____

Please check any of the following that apply:

○ I would be interested in attending a class where I can learn more about spiritual gifts and other factors that God has given me to serve in ministry.

○ I would like to be contacted on how I can become involved in a ministry of the church that would be best suited to my spiritual gift(s).

Sample Healing Service

2001 Presbyterian Parish Nurse Seminar

Forgiveness and Reconciliation: Where Healing Begins

Leader's Version

Plaza Resolana en Santa Fe / Santa Fe, New Mexico

Vespers

Atencio Meeting Room

Thursday, June 28, 2001 / 8:30 - 9:00 p.m.

Keeping the Covenant

Sanctuary and *Shalom* Domestic Violence Healing Prayers

Do no wrong or violence . . .

– Jeremiah 22:3

In silence, prepare your heart and soul for morningsong, prayer, and renewal

PRELUDE–*Day Is Done*–James Quinn

L: The Societal Violence Initiative Team, Violence Against Women, Presbyterian Church (U.S.A.) in 1997 affirmed that . . .

Violence against women is contrary to God's intention for the world. This reality demands the response of the church in these days of increasing danger to women. Interpreting biblical teachings and responding to the leadership of Jesus Christ in our lives, the church is called to a pastoral and moral response through an active program of education, consciousness raising, and empowerment for change.

Vespers for this evening focus on the biblical injunction to *Do no wrong or violence . . .* and to lift up the silent voices of those who live daily in fear or actual violence to themselves and their children. Each one of us has in some way been touched by violence—a family member, a dear friend, ourselves, or someone we have read about in the newspapers.

The sheer breaking of the silence of domestic violence can raise strong emotional responses. If our time together becomes so difficult to bear alone, feel free to leave this sacred space at any time. Also, if you need to talk confidentially with someone during or following morning prayers, you can talk with _____, or myself afterwards.

During our closing hymn, you may come forward to light a candle for someone for whom you are lifting up in prayer today.

OPENING SENTENCES

L: O God, come to our assistance.

P: O Lord, hasten to help us.

L: The Lord our God gives us salvation and victory!

P: The Lord our God brings us light and life!

L: God's right hand has done wonders!

P: So let us proclaim the works of our God!

THE CLOTHESLINE PROJECT

A visual display that bears witness to the violence against women.

L: A visual display that bears witness to the violence against women. The statistics generally are that one in four women are or have been victims of abuse—be it physical, emotional and psychological, economically, and/or sexual. These shirts today have been placed around our sacred space, a silent voice for those with whom we come in contact with every day who experience violence. Each shirt tells a story.

White: Women who have died of violence

Yellow or Beige: Women who have been battered or assaulted

Red, Pink, or Orange: Women who have been raped or sexually assaulted

Blue or Green: Women who are survivors of incest or child sexual abuse

Purple or Lavender: Women attacked because of their sexual orientation

READING

I Got Flowers Today . . . – Author Unknown

PSALTER *(Responsive by verse)*–Psalm 55:4-8, 12–22 REB

L: As you read and listen, hear the voice of one living with violence.

4. My heart is in anguish within me, the terrors of death have fallen upon me,

5. Fear and trembling come upon me, and horror overwhelms me,

6. And I say, "O that I had wings like a dove! I would fly away and be at rest;

7. Truly, I would flee far away; I would lodge in the wilderness;

8. I would hurry to find a shelter for myself from the raging wind and tempest."

12. It is not enemies who taunt me—I could bear that; it is not adversaries who deal insolently with me—I could hide from them.

13. But it is you, my equal, my companion, my familiar friend,

14. With whom I kept pleasant company; we walked in the house of God with the throng.

15. Let death come upon them, let them go down alive in Sheol; for evil is in their homes and in their hearts.

16. But I call upon God, and the Lord will save me.

17. Evening and morning and at noon I utter my complaint and moan, and God will hear my voice.

18. God will redeem me unharmed from the battle that I wage, for many are arrayed against me.

19. God, who is enthroned from of old, will hear, and will humble them—because they do not change, and do not fear God.

20. My companion laid hands on a friend and violated a covenant with me

21. With speech smoother than butter, but with a heart set on war; with words that were softer than oil, but in fact were drawn swords.

22. Cast your burden on the Lord, and God will sustain you; God will never permit the righteous to be moved.

GOSPEL READING – Luke 13:1–17

R: Now listen for the Word of God contained in this story of a woman who may have been a victim of domestic violence . . .

R: Now hear what the Spirit is saying to God's people.

P: Thanks be to God!

(A brief period of silence will be kept)

PRAYERS FOR HEALING – adapted from Caroline Sproul Fairless

L: God of grace, you nurture us with a love deeper than any we know, and your will for us is always healing and salvation.

God of love, you enter into our lives, our pain, and our brokenness, and you stretch out your healing hands to us wherever we are.

God of strength, you fill us with your presence and send us forth with love and healing to all whom we meet.

P: We praise and thank you, O God.

L: God of love, we ask you to hear the prayers of your people.

We pray for the world, that your creation may be understood and valued.

Touch with your healing power the minds and hearts of all who live in confusion or doubt, and fill them with your light.

Touch with your healing power the minds and hearts of all who are burdened by anguish, despair, or isolation, and set them free in love.

P: Hear us, O God of life.

L: Break the bonds of those who are imprisoned by fear, compulsion, secrecy, and silence.

Fill with peace those who grieve over separation and loss.

P: Come with your healing power, O God.

L: Restore to wholeness all those who have been broken in life or in spirit by violence within their families; restore to wholeness all those who have been broken by violence with our Family of Nations, restore to them the power of your love; and give them the strength of your presence.

P: Come, O God, and restore us to wholeness and love.

L: Let us name before God and this community gathered those, including ourselves, for whom we seek healing . . .

(Those gathered may name others silently or out loud)

L: That they may find *sanctuary* and *shalom*.

P: In our homes, our workplaces, our communities, our churches, and in this world.

L: Let us name before God those of this faith community who bear witness of your love and grace . . .

(Those gathered may name others silently or out loud)

L: We lift up before you this day all those who have died of violence . . .

(Those gathered may name others silently or out loud)

L: That they may have rest.

P: In that place where there is no pain or grief, but life eternal.

L: O God, in you all is turned to light, and brokenness is healed. Look with compassion on us and on those for whom we pray, that we may be *re*created in wholeness, in love, and in compassion for one another.

UNISON PRAYER

God of comfort and strength, revive us when we are weary, console us when we are full of woe, and set our feet anew in the way Christ leads us.

Protect us from sin so we may always be glad disciples, diligent in service and bold in witness for our risen Lord, Jesus Christ, Savior of the world. Amen.

THE LORD'S PRAYER

HYMN

> There Is a Balm in Gilead PH 394 – African-American Spiritual
> *(During the singing of this spiritual, those gathered may come forward and light a candle in prayer or memory for an individual for whom they know is living with or has died from violence.)*

DISMISSAL

L: The Psalmist reminds us that . . . *Weeping may linger for the night, but joy comes in the morning.* We have much to be thankful for the work and ministry that has and is being done for those who live with domestic violence. You may be aware that the Advisory Committee on Social Witness Policy document *Turning Mourning into Dancing* was unanimously approved and accepted at the 213th General Assembly in Louisville, Kentucky, just weeks ago. A policy statement contains theological reflection and some 60+ action recommendations for our denomination to take as a stance against domestic violence. In addition, a new network of the Presbyterian Health, Education and Welfare Association *Presbyterians Against Domestic Violence Network* was approved by the PHEWA Biennial in January 2001 and is up and running.

I would be remiss if I also did not mention the effect the work and ministry of Parish Nurses and Health Ministry programs within the lives of congregations have had in raising awareness and prevention education as well as providing initial counsel and guidance with those families whose lives are confronted with domestic violence on a daily basis. We have much to celebrate and be thankful for. Thanks be to God!

L: The grace of God be with us all, now and always.

P: Amen.

L: Bless the Lord.

P: The Lord's name be praised.

> *Ms. Edna Currie, Pianist*
> *Terry Stumpf, Worship Leader*

I got flowers today. And it wasn't . . .

I got flowers today. It wasn't my birthday or any other special day . . .
We had our first argument last night.
And he said a lot of cruel things that really hurt me.
I know he's sorry and didn't mean the things he said . . .
Because he sent me flowers today.
I got flowers today. It wasn't our anniversary or any other special day . . .
Last night, he threw me into a wall and started to choke me.
It seemed like a nightmare.
I couldn't believe it was real.
I woke up this morning sore and bruised all over.
I know he must be sorry . . .
Because he sent me flowers today.
I got flowers today, and it wasn't Mother's Day or any other special day . . .
Last night, he beat me up again.
And it was much worse than all the other times.
If I leave him, what will I do?
How will I take care of my kids? What about money?
But I know he must be sorry . . .
Because he sent me flowers today.
I got flowers today. Lots and lots of flowers. Today was a very special day . . .
It was the day of my funeral.
Last night, he finally killed me.
He beat me to death.
If only I had gathered
enough courage and strength to leave him . . .
I would not have gotten flowers today.

–Author Unknown

Forgiveness and Reconciliation: *Where Healing Begins*

Participant's Version
8:30–9:00 p.m.

Keeping the Covenant
Worship Leader: Dr. Terrill Stumpf *Sanctuary* and *Shalom*
Domestic Violence Healing Prayers

Do no wrong or violence. . . .
– Jeremiah 22:3

In silence, prepare your heart and soul for evensong, prayer, and renewal

PRELUDE – *Day Is Done* – James Quinn

OPENING SENTENCES •

L: O God, come to our assistance.
P: O Lord, hasten to help us.
L: The Lord our God gives us salvation and victory!
P: The Lord our God brings us light and life!
L: God's right hand has done wonders!
P: So let us proclaim the works of our God!

THE CLOTHESLINE PROJECT

A visual display that bears witness to the violence against women.
White: Women who have died of violence
Yellow or Beige: Women who have been battered or assaulted
Red, Pink, or Orange: Women who have been raped or sexually
assaulted
Blue or Green: Women who are survivors of incest or child sexual
abuse
Purple or Lavender: Women attacked because of their sexual
orientation

READING

I Got Flowers Today . . . – Author Unknown

PSALTER *(Responsive by verse)* – Psalm 55:4-8, 12–22 REB

4. My heart is in anguish within me, the terrors of death have fallen
upon me,

5. Fear and trembling come upon me, and horror overwhelms me,

6. And I say, "O that I had wings like a dove! I would fly away and be at rest;

7. Truly, I would flee far away; I would lodge in the wilderness;

8. I would hurry to find a shelter for myself from the raging wind and tempest."

12. It is not enemies who taunt me—I could bear that; it is not adversaries who deal insolently with me—I could hide from them.

13. But it is you, my equal, my companion, my familiar friend,

14. With whom I kept pleasant company; we walked in the house of God with the throng.

15. Let death come upon them, let them go down alive in Sheol; for evil is in their homes and in their hearts.

16. But I call upon God, and the Lord will save me.

17. Evening and morning and at noon I utter my complaint and moan, and God will hear my voice.

18. God will redeem me unharmed from the battle that I wage, for many are arrayed against me.

19. God, who is enthroned from of old, will hear, and will humble them—because they do not change, and do not fear God.

20. My companion laid hands on a friend and violated a covenant with me

21. With speech smoother than butter, but with a heart set on war; with words that were softer than oil, but in fact were drawn swords.

22. Cast your burden on the Lord, and God will sustain you; God will never permit the righteous to be moved.   ❀

GOSPEL READING Luke 13:1–17
R: Now hear what the Spirit is saying to God's people.
P: Thanks be to God!
(A brief period of silence will be kept.)

PRAYERS FOR HEALING – adapted from Caroline Sproul Fairless
L: God of grace, you nurture us with a love deeper than any we know, and your will for us is always healing and salvation.

God of love, you enter into our lives, our pain, and our brokenness, and you stretch out your healing hands to us wherever we are.

God of strength, you fill us with your presence and send us forth with love and healing to all whom we meet.
P: We praise and thank you, O God.

L: God of love, we ask you to hear the prayers of your people.

We pray for the world, that your creation may be understood and valued.

Touch with your healing power the minds and hearts of all who live in confusion or doubt, and fill them with your light.

Touch with your healing power the minds and hearts of all who are burdened by anguish, despair, or isolation, and set them free in love.

P: Hear us, O God of life.

L: Break the bonds of those who are imprisoned by fear, compulsion, secrecy, and silence.

Fill with peace those who grieve over separation and loss.

P: Come with your healing power, O God.

L: Restore to wholeness all those who have been broken in life or in spirit by violence within their families; restore to wholeness all those who have been broken by violence with our Family of Nations, restore to them the power of your love; and give them the strength of your presence.

P: Come, O God, and restore us to wholeness and love.

L: Let us name before God and this community gathered those, including ourselves, for whom we seek healing . . .

(Those gathered may name others silently or out loud)

L: That they may find *sanctuary* and *shalom*.

P: In our homes, our workplaces, our communities, our churches, and in this world.

L: Let us name before God those of this faith community who bear witness of your love and grace . . .

(Those gathered may name others silently or out loud)

L: We lift up before you this day all those who have died of violence . . .

(Those gathered may name others silently or out loud)

L: That they may have rest.

P: In that place where there is no pain or grief, but life eternal.

L: O God, in you all is turned to light, and brokenness is healed. Look with compassion on us and on those for whom we pray, that we may be *re*created in wholeness, in love, and in compassion for one another.

UNISON PRAYER

God of comfort and strength, revive us when we are weary, console us when we are full of woe, and set our feet anew in the way Christ leads us. Protect us from sin so we may always be glad disciples, diligent in service and bold in witness for our risen Lord, Jesus Christ, Savior of the world. Amen.

THE LORD'S PRAYER

HYMN

There Is a Balm in Gilead PH 394– African-American Spiritual

(During the singing of this spiritual, those gathered may come forward and light a candle in prayer or memory for an individual for whom they know is living with or has died from violence.)

DISMISSAL

L: The grace of God be with us all, now and always.

P: Amen.

L: Bless the Lord.

P: The Lord's name be praised.

Notes

PREFACE

1. Carson, V. B. (1989). *Spiritual dimensions of nursing practice.* Philadelphia: W. B. Saunders, pp. 55–56.

2. McNamara, K. (Spring/Summer, 2000). *Remembered forever. Perspectives in parish nursing practice.* Park Ridge, IL: Advocate Health Care, p. 12. This is a tribute to Rev. Westberg written by his granddaughter. He died on Tuesday, February 16, 1999.

3. Health Ministries Association and American Nurses Association. (1998). *Scope and standards of parish nursing practice.* Washington, DC: American Nurses Publishing, p. 1.

I. RESPONDING TO THE CALL

1. Thanks to Father William Franken, pastor of St. John the Evangelist Church in Hydes, Maryland. One of us (VBC) had been praying about chapter 1, asking for God's guidance. On May 6, Father Willie (as he is affectionately called) gave a wonderful sermon on hearing and responding to the unique voice of God.

2. Shelly, J. A., and Miller, A. B. (1999). *Called to care: A Christian theology of nursing.* Downers Grove, IL: Intervarsity Press. In chapter 13, "Nursing as a Christian Calling," Shelly and Miller discuss the history of nursing and provide examples of how some of the earliest Catholic nuns and Protestant deaconesses served as nurses not as a commitment to a professional discipline but as a response to God's call to service.

3. Karaban, R. A. (1998). *Responding to God's call: A survival guide.* San Jose, CA: Resource Publications, Inc., p. 15.

4. Ibid., pp. 3–4.

5. Marianne Parker is the parish nursing program coordinator for St. Joseph's Hospital in Syracuse, New York. Marianne has developed creative programs for use by the parish nurses whom she supervises. Marianne can be reached at marianne.parker@sjhsyr.org or St. Joseph's Hospital-Congregational Health; Attn: Marianne E. Parker, RN, 301 Prospect Avenue, Syracuse, NY 13203.

6. Carole Kornelis is a parish nurse for First Reformed Church located at 6th and Grover Streets, Lynden, WA 98262; telephone: 260-354-4221. E-mail: VanderKooiC@lynden.wednet.edu.

7. Susan Dyess is a parish nurse in Florida. She has served in two paid positions—one hospital based, the other academically based.

8. Catherine Lomax serves as a parish nurse at the Church of the Good Samaritan in Paoli, Pennsylvania.

9. Ellen Altenhofer participated in a "Called to Care" seminar held in Plymouth Congregational Church in Washington State. This program served as the foundation for the parish nurse program that became part of the church constitution in the fall of 1995. Ellen served as the parish care coordinator until September 1996, when she was joined in this effort by Joan Wieringa. In January 1999, Ellen stepped down from the role of parish care coordinator, although she continues to serve as a parish nurse in the capacity of parish care committee resource member.

10. Pauline Sheehan is a parish nurse in Everett, Washington. In 1998, Pauline wrote a book entitled *Hugs for Caregivers* (Enumclaw, WA: Wine Press Pub.).

11. Rose S. Young is the parish nurse at New Virginia United Methodist Church in Hermitage, Pennsylvania.

12. Barb McDonald of Redmond, Washington, had a dream to start the "Dream Team" in her church. From her experience with the "Dream Team" she became the parish nurse, a position that goes hand in hand with the work of the "Dream Team."

13. Twadell, A. S. (Fall/Winter, 1999). Personal perspective. *Perspectives in parish nursing practice.* Park Ridge, IL: Advocate Health Care, pp. 7, 9.

14. Matheus, R. (Fall/Winter, 2000). Personal perspective. *Perspectives in parish nursing practice.* Park Ridge, IL, Advocate Health Care, pp. 6–7. When Rosemarie was contacted regarding sharing her story, she generously created an audio tape that provides rich details regarding her role as teacher to parish nurses. This tape is referred to in other chapters of this book.

15. Griffin, J. (Spring/Summer, 2000). Personal perspective. *Perspectives in parish nursing practice.* Park Ridge, IL: Advocate Health Care, pp. 7–8.

16. Martin, L. B. (January 1996). Parish nursing: keeping body and soul together. *The Canadian Nurse,* 25–28. In this article Linda B. Martin (now Dr. Lynda W. Miller) describes the evolution of the parish nurse movement in Canada. The First Lutheran Church in Vancouver adopted Granger Westberg's health center model in the early 1980s. The Vancouver Center functioned for eighteen months and disbanded owing to outside job commitments of the pastor and physician. The nurse member of the team, Grace Hodgins, says that if she had known then what she knows now (in 1996) she would have continued solo and become Canada's first parish nurse. This may be an example of God laying a foundation for the future. The growth of parish nursing in Canada has taken a different course than what has occurred in the United States. There were no educational programs to prepare parish nurses in Canada until Inter-Church Health Ministries developed classes in October 1995 for six parish nurses in a pilot project in Oshawa, Ontario. The project developed from the seed planted in 1994 by nurses Maureen MacLeod and Carol Crossman, who had received a $10,000 Healthy Communities grant from the

Ontario Ministry of Health. The faculty of nursing of the University of Alberta in Edmonton began to offer a thirteen-session preparation course in 1996. Many of the earliest Canadian parish nurses were educated through programs in the United States. The author completed a program in 1993 in Portland, Oregon. She was followed a year later by a colleague, Patricia O'Meara-Thompson, who went on to develop a health assessment and referral role within her congregation's pastoral care committee that focused on the care of frail elderly parishioners. Dawn Dyer, another Canadian parish nurse pioneer, of Peterborough, Ontario, completed a parish nurse program sponsored by Mercy Hospital in Grayling, Michigan. Dyer held a half-time position as a member of the pastoral staff of her diocese. She conducted a survey of parishioners' needs. This survey led her to develop a range of health promotion activities including a health fair, a CPR course, a newsletter, and nutrition counseling. In May 1995, the author initiated a BC Forum—New Perspectives on Health Promotion Ministries in Churches—was co-sponsored by Trinity Western University and Nurses Christian Fellowship. Five parish nurses from Oregon and Washington State came to Langley, British Columbia, to share their knowledge with Canadian nurses. A representative from the Registered Nurses Association of British Columbia also participated and dialogue began regarding standards for courses and practice.

17. Miller, L.W. (Winter, 1997). Nursing through the lens of faith: a conceptual model. *Journal of Christian Nursing, 14 (1),* 17–20. In this article Lynda describes her own journey into parish nursing and provides an overview of the general nursing theoretical framework she developed to undergird the practice from a clearly Christian worldview. An in-depth description is presented in her doctoral dissertation, "A Nursing Conceptual Model Grounded in Christian Faith," University of Victoria, BC (1996). Her e-mail is lwmiller@attcanada.net.

18. Kelly Preston is the congregational health program coordinator for the Ingalls Center of Pastoral Ministries, Baptist Health System of Alabama. The Baptist Health System shares a mission statement that seems appropriate for any congregation offering a health-care ministry. The mission statement is "As a witness to the love of God revealed through Jesus Christ, the Baptist Health System is committed to ministries that enhance the health, dignity, and wholeness of those we serve, through integrity, compassion, advocacy, resourcefulness, and excellence." Kelly shares a Model for Ministry that she developed and that guides her work. The model is discussed later in chapter 7. Kelly's e-mail address is Kelly.Preston@ BHSALA.com; telephone: 205-783-3495.

19. Dianne Smith served as a parish nurse for three years before feeling the call to plant nurses in churches. She believes that she serves God by serving parish nurses, who in turn serve others. Dianne ministers in southern Florida and is based in Orlando. Her e-mail address is DparishNrs@aol.com; telephone: 407-282-9655.

20. Schutte, Dan. (1994). Here I am, Lord. In Robert J. Batastini and Michael A. Cymbala (Eds.), *Gather* (2nd ed.), (Hymn 492). Chicago: GIA Publications, Inc.

2. CALLED TO SERVE:
MINISTRY OF WORD AND ACTION

1. Griffin, J. (Spring/Summer, 2000). Personal perspective. *Perspectives in parish nursing practice.* Park Ridge, IL: Advocate Health Care), p. 7.

2. Westberg, Granger. (1987). *The parish nurse: How to start a parish nurse program in your church.* Park Ridge, IL: Parish Nurse Resource Center), pp. 8–9.

3. Holstrom, S. (1999). Perspectives on a suburban practice. In Phyllis Ann Solari-Twadell and Mary Ann McDermott (Eds.), *Parish nursing: Promoting whole person health within faith communities* (pp. 69–73). Thousand Oaks, CA: Sage Publications, Inc. Clark, M. B., and Olson, J. K. (2000). *Nursing within a faith community: Promoting health in times of transition,* pp. 141–154. Thousand Oaks, CA: Sage Publications, Inc.

4. Sensenig, J. (1993). *Nurse in the congregation: A guidebook for planning health ministries in Mennonite churches,* 3. (Published by the author: New Holland, PA, 1044 Ranck Road).

5. Dianne Smith is a parish nursing consultant and educator in Orlando, Florida. Her e-mail address is DparishNrs@aol.com.

6. Koenig, H. (2001). Presented at the conference "Faith in the future: Religion, aging, and healthcare in the 21st century," Duke University, Durham, North Carolina, March 4.

7. Swinney, J., Anson-Wonkka, C., Maki, E., and Corneau, J. (January–February 2001). Community assessment: A church community and the parish nurse. *Public Health Nursing, 18 (1),* 40–44.

8. This information came from the following sources. Rose S. Young, from her parish nursing report of February, 2001 to the New Virginia United Methodist Church in Hermitage, Pennsylvania. Kelly Preston's story of her role as congregational health program coordinator of Baptist Health System in Alabama contained many helpful ideas. Pruski, Thomas. (August 10, 2000). Our congregations—where physical and spiritual health can prevail. *The Catholic Standard. The Catholic Standard* is a publication of the Archdiocese of Washington, DC. Tom is the health and wellness coordinator of Wellness Works–Catholic Charities of Montgomery County. Visit Tom's web site at www.wellworks.org, or e-mail pruskit@catholiccharities-dc.org, or phone 301-942-1856 (ext. 109). Marianne Parker shared the results of a survey conducted by St. Joseph's Hospital Congregational Health Program and summarized over four thousand health promotion contacts and two thousand hours of volunteer time donated to the twenty-nine churches active in the program, the five churches that are forming a congregational health ministry, and the fifteen churches that are interested in forming a congregational ministry!

9. Buijs, R., and Olson, J. (2001). Parish nurses influencing determinants of health. *Journal of Community Health Nursing, 18 (1),* 13–23.

10. Ellen Altenhofer was a parish nurse at Normandy Park Congregational Church, 413 SW 197th St., Seattle, WA 98166; 206-824-39876. In June 1999, Ellen stepped down from the position of parish nurse coordinator but she has continued

to support the health ministry in her church as a parish care committee resource member. Joan Wieringa shared the position of parish nurse coordinator with Ellen and now has continued in the role of coordinator—a role that became a paid position in January 1999.

11. Deborah Baker, RN, B.S.N., is a parish nurse at First Presbyterian Church in Petaluma, CA. Deborah's e-mail address is DebPHN@aol.com.

12. Marianne Parker is the congregational health program coordinator for St. Joseph's Hospital Health Center in Syracuse, NY.

13. Smith, S., Freeland, M., Heffler, S., McKusick, D., and The Health Expenditures Projection Team. (1998). The next ten years of health spending: What does the future hold? *Health Affairs, 17,* 128–140.

14. Parker, Marianne. (Summer, 2000). Mobilizing volunteers for service. *Healing Hearts and Hands, 4 (3),* 1. This is a publication edited by Marianne Parker. The publication is an example of the teaching/communication resources developed by parish nurses. In this particular issue, Marianne discusses how to mobilize volunteers; examines the sources of tension and provides wholistic suggestions to deal with tension; provides a calendar of upcoming community events; announces upcoming seminars and networking opportunities for parish nurses; shares stories of parish nurses; discusses prayer requests; highlights vision research as well as vision for ministry—both requiring periodic examination; and makes suggestions for parish nurses to support biblical parenting.

15. Oman, D., Thoresen, C., and McMahon, K. (1999). Volunteerism and mortality among the community-dwelling elderly. *Journal of Health Psychology, 4 (3),* 301–316. Freedman, M. (1999). *Prime time: How baby boomers will revolutionize retirement and transform America.* New York: Public Affairs. Koenig, H. G. (2002). *Purpose and power in retirement.* Philadelphia, PA: Templeton Foundation Press.

16. Parker, 1.

17. Gaul, C. (June 21, 2001). If you ask them, they will come. *The Catholic Review, 67 (10),* 1, 3.

18. Parker, 1.

19. Judy Shelly also discusses the role of the parish nurse in organizing and coordinating groups to serve in health-related areas such as prayer chains, home visitation, and providing meals for the sick.

20. Catherine Lomax is a parish nurse at the Church of the Good Samaritan located at 212 West Lancaster Avenue in Paoli, PA 19301. The telephone number is 610-644-4040 ext. 223.

21. Buijs and Olson, 13–23.

22. Carole Kornelis is the parish nurse at First Reformed Church located at 6th and Grover Street, Lynden, WA 260-354-4221. Carole works and is supported by the Reverend Marc deWaard.

23. Parker, 1.

24. Kelly Preston is congregational health program coordinator at the Ingalls Center of Pastoral Ministries of the Baptist Health Care System of Alabama. Kelly

can be reached at Princeton Baptist Medical Center, 701 Princeton Avenue, Birmingham, AL 35211-1399.

25. Joyce McCasland, a parish nurse at a Catholic church in Minnesota can be reached by e-mail at Joyce@mccaslands.com

26. Cheryl Hovland is a parish nurse for MeritCare Healthcare in Pelican Rapids, Minnesota., She can be reached at cherylhovland2@meritcare.com.

27. Palmer, Jane. (First quarter, 2001). Parish nursing: Connecting faith and health. *Reflections on Nursing Leadership,* 17–19.

28. Susan Dyess is a parish nurse coordinator and educator at Atlantic University in Boca Raton, Florida and St. Mary's Hospital in West Palm Beach, Florida.

3. THE JOURNEY OF THE PARISH NURSE WITHIN THE CHURCH

1. Carson, V. B. (2000). *Mental health nursing: The nurse-patient journey (2nd ed.).* Philadelphia: W.B. Saunders and Company, p. 3.

2. Dianne Smith is a parish nurse consultant and educator in south Florida; she can be reached by e-mail at DparishNrs@aol.com.

3. Kristine Holmes was quoting Dahl, M. (Spring, 1994). Watch for G.M.C.'s. *Great is his love.* Moline, IL: Trinity Medical Center.

4. Kristine Holmes, RN, B.S., is a parish nurse at First Presbyterian Church of Howard County in Columbia, Maryland. Kris has been in this position for five years. She worked in an unpaid position from 1996 to 1999. Beginning in 2000 Kris assumed a full-time paid position. She is also involved in identifying existing and emerging parish nurse/health ministries in Howard County, Maryland. She has now coordinated the growing network in Howard County—with monthly meetings. These meetings involve a time of devotions, networking, case presentations, and special programs. On alternate months the special program either focuses on existing county agencies and services or on spiritual growth and development to better equip nurses to spiritual care. Kristine can be reached at kris@1stpreshc.org.

5. Anna Friedberg is the coordinator of the health ministry team at a small church in East Syracuse, New York; she can be reached at 315-448-2773.

6. Karen Thornton is the parish nurse at St. Mark the Evangelist Catholic Church in Grand Blanc, Michigan; her e-mail address is thornzinger@aol.com.

7. Ellen Kirker is the coordinator of the Congregational Health Ministry at Holy Spirit Hospital in Camp Hill, Pennsylvania. This is a paid position that was originally funded by a grant from the Robert Wood Johnson Foundation but is now solely supported by hospital monies. The program has an ecumenical focus.

8. Maddox, M. (2001). Circle of Christian caring: a model for parish nursing practice. *Journal of Christian Nursing, 18 (3),* 11–13.

9. Linda Whitesell is a parish nurse at Prince of Peace Lutheran Church in Everett, Washington.

10. Marianne Parker currently serves as the coordinator of the Parish Nurse Program sponsored by St. Joseph's Hospital in Syracuse, New York.

11. Dr. Ruth Stoll, RN, CS-P, is a parish nurse in Pennsylvania. She began her journey by developing a certification course for parish nurses that was offered at Messiah College. She taught this course from the early 1990s until she retired in 1996. She began by working in her own Presbyterian Church in an unpaid capacity. In 1992, she became the parish nurse at the Episcopal Cathedral in Harrisburg, Pennsylvania. Dr. Stoll can be reached at ris15@juno.com.

12. Debbie Hyder is a parish nurse at Bethel Presbyterian USA in Kingston, Tennessee. Debbie was commissioned as a parish nurse on Easter Sunday, 1999.

13. Carole Kornelis is a parish nurse in Washington State. Her e-mail address is VanderKooiC@lynden.webnet.edu.

14. Shelly, J. A. (Winter, 1997). Working toward shalom. *Journal of Christian Nursing, 14 (1),* 3. Dr. Judy Shelly is an author and parish nurse at St. Luke's Lutheran Church in Obelisk, Pennsylvania.

15. Catherine Lick, RN, M.S.N., is a paid parish nurse at Faith Lutheran Church in Troy, Michigan.

16. Catherine Lomax, RN, serves as a parish nurse at the Church of the Good Samaritan in Paoli, Pennsylvania.

17. Ibid.

18. Karen Thornton, RN, is an unpaid parish nurse at St. Mark's Evangelist Catholic Church in Grand Blanc, Michigan.

19. Terrill Stumpf, RN, DNSc, is the director of Health Ministry at the Fourth Presbyterian Church of Chicago. He was a seminarian at McCormack Theological Seminary in Chicago and served as a parish nurse at Old Presbyterian Church in San Francisco. He is involved in Domestic Violence Awareness as a ministry of the Presbyterian Church (U.S.A.). Terry's e-mail address: tstumpf@fourthchurch.org.

20. Kelly Preston is the coordinator of the Congregational Health Program for the Ingalls Center of Pastoral Ministries, Baptist Health System of Alabama. Her e-mail address is Kelly.Preston@BHSALA.com; and her telephone number is 205-783-3495.

4. THE JOURNEY INTO THE COMMUNITY

1. Tom Pruski is the coordinator of Wellness Works. The website is www.wellworks.org.

2. Dr. Ruth Stoll is a parish nurse educator and consultant in central Pennsylvania. She was a professor of psychiatric nursing at Messiah College in Pennsylvania until she retired in 1996. She then assumed a part-time paid parish nurse position at St. Stephen's Episcopal Cathedral in Harrisburg. She began in 1996 working ten hours per week, gradually increasing her time commitment to more than twenty hours per week. In 2000, she felt called by God to focus her energies on the development of lay health ministers in the African-American churches. Dr. Stoll is a

sought-after educator in the northeast area of the country. She regularly teaches the spiritual component of the endorsed parish nurse curriculum when the course is offered in Pennsylvania. She is active on the Presbyterian Parish Nurse Task Force. Her e-mail address is ris15@juno.com

3. Maggie Spielman's story is quoted in Singer, N. (2001). Parish nursing: Jesus people style. *Journal of Christian Nursing, 18 (3),* 5–7. Used with permission.

4. Kristine Holmes is a parish nurse at First Presbyterian Church of Howard County in Columbia, Maryland. The video that Kristine refers to presents the stories of four women who have been victims of domestic violence. Two of the women are from the Protestant tradition, one is Roman Catholic, and the other is Jewish. After these women present their stories, clergy from each faith tradition respond. The video is available from the Center for the Prevention of Sexual and Domestic Violence, 2400 N. 45th St. #10, Seattle, WA 98103; 206-636-1903; Kristine's e-mail address is: kris@1stpreshc.org.

5. The Clothesline Project is a visual display of shirts designed by women survivors of violence and family/friends of women victims of violence. The project bears witness to the violence against women, educates the public, and provides active solutions for violence prevention. Terry has used resources from The Clothesline Project in Chicago, located at 12627 W. 143rd Street, Lockport, IL, 60441; 704-645-0798; www.clothesline.org; as well as The Clothesline Project located in Jicarilla Mental Health and Social Services in Dulce, New Mexico 87528; 1-800-942-7440.

6. Terrill L. Stumpf, RN, DNSc, is the director of Health Ministry at Fourth Presbyterian Church in Chicago, Illinois. Terry has extensive background in nursing practice, administration, and education. He was a writer and part of the panel that revised the Parish Nurse Education Curricula (2000) through the International Parish Nurse Resource Center, Park Ridge, Illinois. A copy of this worship service—for the participant as well as for the leader—is found in Appendix B. Dr. Stumpf also used this same worship at the 2001 Presbyterian Parish Nurse Seminar held at Plaza Resolana in Sante Fe, New Mexico.

7. Cooney, Rory. (1994). Jerusalem, my destiny. In Robert J. Batastini and Michael A. Cymbala (Eds.), *Gather* (2nd ed.). Chicago, IL: GIA Publications, Inc.

5 . PREPARATION FOR THE JOURNEY

1. Quindlen, Anna. (2000). *A short guide to a happy life.* New York: Random House.

2. Albom, Mitch. (1997). *Tuesdays with Morrie.* New York: Doubleday.

3. McCormick, Patrick. (2001). Pass it on. *U.S. Catholic, 66 (8),* 46–48.

4. *Journal of Christian Nursing* published this interview with Granger Westberg in its Winter 1989 issue. The interviewer's name was not given. Parish nursing's pioneer: A *JCN* interview with Granger Westberg. *Journal of Christian Nursing, 6 (1),* 26–29.

5. Ann Solari-Twadell is the former director of the International Parish Nurse Resource Center.

6. Solari-Twadell, P. A., and McDermott, M. A. (1999). *Parish nursing: Promoting whole person health within faith communities.* Thousand Oaks, CA: Sage Press, pp. 269–275.

7. Rosemarie Matheus is a recognized leader in the education of parish nurses and in the development of new parish nurse programs. She provides parish nurse education across the country and serves as a consultant to individual parish nurses and congregations interested in developing parish nurse programs. Rosemarie can be reached at JTMRM@aol.com.

8. Norma Small RN, Ph.D., CRNP, serves as a consultant for Health Ministries Association (HMA), a membership organization for those involved in health ministries, including parish nurses. Norma runs her own consulting business, Concerned Care Management and Consultation, Inc. She offers a course in parish nursing entitled Concepts and Practice of Parish Nursing and Health Ministries. The address of her consultation firm is 1077 Crest Avenue, Johnstown, PA 15902; telephone and fax #: 814-539-2273; e-mail address: nrsmall@aol.com.

9. Dr. Ruth Stoll, formerly a professor of psychiatric nursing at Messiah College, is now retired from teaching but involved full time as a parish nurse educator and consultant. Her current ministry focus is the development of lay health ministries within African-American Churches in Pennsylvania. See chapter 4 for further discussion of this ministry.

10. Health Ministries Association (HMA). (1998). *The scope and standards of parish nursing practice.* Washington, DC: American Nurses Association. This document is available from the ANA by calling 800-637-0323. The publication number is 9806STCM2; the cost is $14.95 plus shipping and handling.

11. Carol Story is the director of Puget Sound Parish Nurse Ministries. She can be reached at carolms@msn.com.

12. Sandra Thomas, M.Div., D.Min., is the director of Partners in Parish Nursing. She can be reached at Partners in Parish Nursing, 450 Ski Lane, Millersville, MD 21108-1995; 410-729-5672 or 1-800-732-5672; fax: 410-729-5674; or e-mail: Learn@Partners-ParishNursing.org.

13. The Reverend Donna Coffman is a nurse and an ordained minister in the Presbyterian Church. She teaches a course called Caring Congregations at Union Theological Seminary and Presbyterian School of Christian Education in Richmond, Virginia. She can be reached at dcoffman@union.psce.edu or 804-254-8070. Donna also served as chairperson of the Presbyterian Parish Nurse Task Force and in this position coordinated several national conferences for parish nurses. One is held in Sante Fe, New Mexico, at Plaza Resolana and the other at Stony Point, New York, two of the three national conference and retreat centers of the Presbyterian Church (USA).

1. Shelly, J. A. and Miller, A. B. (1999). *Called to care: A Christian theology of nursing*. Downers Grove, IL: Intervarsity Press.

2. *Journal of Christian Nursing* published this interview with Granger Westberg in its Winter 1989 issue. The interviewer's name was not given. Parish nursing's pioneer: A *JCN* interview with Granger Westberg. *Journal of Christian Nursing, 6 (1)*, 26–29.

3. Westberg, Granger. (1987). *The parish nurse: How to start a parish nurse program in your church*. Park Ridge, IL: Parish Nurse Resource Center, pp. 8–9.

4. Health Ministries Association, Inc., and American Nurses Association. (1998). *Scope and standards of parish nursing practice*. Washington, DC: American Nurses Publishing.

5. Remsen, J. (August 5, 2001). A pioneering Jewish "congregational" nurse offers holistic care: Ministering to the body and soul. *Philadelphia Inquirer.*

6. Koenig, H. (2001). Presented at the conference "Faith in the future: Religion, aging and healthcare in the 21st century," Duke University, Durham, North Carolina, March 4.

7. Dr. Linda Scott is a nurse educator at Concordia College in Moorhead, Minnesota, and a member of Evangelical Lutheran Church of America. She lives in Fargo, North Dakota. She can be reached at 218-299-4063 (work) or at lscott@cord.net.

8. Rosemarie Matheus, the director of the Parish Nurse Preparation Institute at Marquette University College of Nursing, shared her insights regarding parish nursing in a taped interview that she graciously made for this book in the spring of 2001.

9. Striepe, J. M., and King, J. M. (Winter, 1993). Basics of beginning a parish nurse program. *Journal of Christian Nursing,* 14–17. Maddox, M. (Summer, 2001). Circle of Christian caring: A model for parish nursing practice. *Journal of Christian Nursing,* 11–13.

10. Miller, L. W. (1997). Nursing through the lens of faith: A conceptual model. *Journal of Christian Nursing, 14 (1),* 17–20.

11. Koenig, "Faith in the future."

12. Smith, Sybil D. (Spring, 1999). Response to God's life-giving ways by Ralph Underwood. *Insights, 14* (2), 29–32. *Insights* is published by the Austin Presbyterian Seminary in Austin, Texas.

13. Boario, Maria T. (Winter, 1993). Mercy model: Church-based health care in the inner city. *Journal of Christian Nursing,* 21–23.

1. Striepe, J. M. and King, J. M. (1993). Basics for beginning a parish nurse program. *Journal of Christian Nursing, 10 (1),* 17.

2. Westberg, Granger. (1990). *The Parish Nurse.* Minneapolis: Augsburg Fortress Press.

3. Dr. Judith Shelly is not only a parish nurse at St. Luke's Lutheran Church in Obelisk, Pennsylvania, she is the editor of the *Journal of Christian Nursing* and the author of many publications.

4. Marianne Parker, RN, is the coordinator of the Parish Nursing Program for St. Joseph's Hospital in Syracuse, New York. Marianne has developed creative programs for use by the parish nurses whom she supervises. Marianne can be reached at marianne.parker@sjhsyr.org or St. Joseph's Hospital-Congregational Health; Attn: Marianne E. Parker, RN, 301 Prospect Avenue, Syracuse, NY 13203. Her telephone number is 315-445-0915.

5. Sagrid E. Edman, RN, Ph.D., was the former chair of the nursing department at Bethel College in St. Paul, Minnesota. In August of 1997, Dr. Edman took the parish nurse preparation course given by Rosemarie Matheus at Marquette University. At the end of the fall semester of 1997, Dr. Edman retired from her faculty position. She felt that parish nursing "fit" with what she believed God wanted her to do in her retirement; it "fit" with her perspective on nursing as a compassionate, caring, and healing ministry; and it "fit" with her years as a nursing educator. Her call has led her to participate as a member of the initial planning group for a parish nurse position and ministry in a church that she eventually joined; to serve as a member of the Parish Nurse Commission of the Northwest Conference of the Evangelical Covenant Church; and to serve as a member and as the chair of the health ministry team in her own church.

6. Dr. Linda Scott is a nurse educator at Concordia College in Moorhead, Minnesota, and a member of Evangelical Lutheran Church of America. She lives in Fargo, North Dakota. She can be reached at 218-299-4063 (work) or at lscott@cord.net.

7. Carole Kornelis is a parish nurse for First Reformed Church located at 6th and Grover Streets, Lynden, WA 98262. The program is affiliated with St. Joseph's Hospital (telephone: 260-354-4221). Carole's e-mail address is VanderKooiC@lynden.wednet.edu. The video that Carole refers to was produced by the Bay Area Health Ministries.

8. Catherine Lomax is the parish nurse at the Church of the Good Samaritan located at 212 West Lancaster Avenue in Paoli, PA 19301. Her telephone number is 610-644-4040 ext 223.

9. Donna Benning is a parish nurse in Bellingham, Washington.

10. Kelly Preston is the coordinator of the Congregational Health Program for the Ingalls Center of Pastoral Ministries, Baptist Health System of Alabama. Kelly

started as a parish nurse before assuming the position of coordinator. She presented the "Preston Congregational Health Program Model for Ministry" on March 5, 2001 at the "Faith in the Future" conference held at Duke University in Durham, North Carolina. Kelly can be reached at Kelly.Preston@BHSALA.com.

8.LOOKING TO THE FUTURE: THE NEXT GENERATION OF PARISH NURSING

1. Health Ministries Association (HMA). (1998). *The scope and standards of parish nursing practice.* Washington, DC: American Nurses Association. This document is available from the ANA by calling 800-637-0323. The publication number is 9806STCM2; the cost is $14.95 plus shipping and handling. This document is scheduled for review in 2003 under the leadership of the co-authors: ANA and HMA. The HMA is the membership organization for those people who serve in the faith health ministry movement; it is recognized by the American Nurses Association as the professional specialty organization for parish nurses and as such has been accepted by the American Nurses Association for membership in the Nursing Organization Liaison Forum (NOLF). Parish nurses make up the largest percentage of HMA members.

2. For more information about the long range activities for nurses within the faith health ministry movement, contact Peggy Matteson, chair of the Practice and Education Committee at 401-683-7475 or peggymatteson@home.com.

3. Shelly, J. A. (2001). Parish nursing: Firing the imagination. An editorial. *Journal of Christian Nursing, 18 (3)*, 3.

4. Ibid.

5. Magilvy, J. K., and Brown, N. J. (1997). Parish nursing: advanced practice nursing. Model for healthier communities. *Advanced Practice Nursing Quarterly, 2 (4)*, 67–72.

6. www.nursing.duke.edu.

7. Chase-Ziolke, M. (1999). The meaning and experience of health ministry within the culture of a congregation with a parish nurse. *Journal of Transcultural Nursing, 10 (1)*, 46–55.

8. Chase-Ziolke, M., and Striepe. J. (1999). A comparison of urban versus rural experiences of nurses volunteering to promote health in churches. *Public Health Nursing, 16 (4)*, 270–279.

9. Chase-Ziolke, M., and Gruca, J. (2000). Client's perceptions of distinctive aspects in nursing care within a congregational setting. *Journal of Community Health Nursing, 17 (3)*, 171–183.

10. Coenen, A., Weis, D. M., Schank, M.J., and Matheus, R. (1999). Describing parish nurse practice using the Nursing Minimum Data Set. *Public Health Nursing, 16 (6)*, 412–416.

References

Abbott, B. (April 1998). Ask home healthcare nurse; parish nursing. *Home Healthcare Nurse, 16 (4)*, 265–267.

Many faith communities have begun offering aid through parish nursing. The parish nurse is a part of the church's or synagogue's ministry to its members and the community at large. Parish nurses are registered nurses, but unlike home care nurses they do not do "hands-on nursing" or bill for their services. Rather, they nurture and support persons in difficult health-related situations. The parish nurse is the safety net needed in an increasingly complex medical system, and promotes wellness physically, socially, emotionally, and spiritually.

Albom, M. (1997). *Tuesdays with Morrie.* New York: Doubleday.

Armmer, F. A., and Humbles, P. (1995). Parish nursing: Extending health care to urban African Americans. *Nursing and Health Care Perspectives on Community, 16 (2)*, 64–68.

Atkins, F. D. (1997). What should the church do about health? A congregational survey. *Journal of Christian Nursing, 14 (1)*, 29–31.

Bay, M. J. (1997). Healing partners: The oncology nurse and the parish nurse. *Seminars in Oncology Nursing, 13 (4)*, 275–278.

The article examines the overlap between the roles of the parish nurse and the oncology nurse and concludes that they can become partners to provide care to patients and their families.

Berquist, S., and King, J. (1994). Parish Nursing—A conceptual framework. *Journal of Holistic Nursing, 12 (2)*, 155–170.

The article describes the roles of the parish nurse and how these roles fit into a conceptual framework of five broad categories of client, health, nurse, environment, and nursing practice. These five categories provide a framework for organizing the concept of parish nursing for future nursing theory, research, and practice.

Biddix, V., and Brown, H. N. Establishing a parish nurse program. *Nursing and Health Care Perspectives, 20 (2)*, 72–75.

This article describes the establishment of a program in an 800-member Baptist church in a city of 66,700, located in a mountainous county of western North Carolina. The authors worked with the team that set up the program.

Blazer, D. G., Landerman, L.R., Fillenbaum, G., and Horner, R. (1995). Health services access and use among older adults in North Carolina: Urban vs. rural residents. *American Journal of Public Health, 85 (10),* 1384–1390.

Boario, M. T. (1993). Mercy model: Church-based health care in the inner city. *Church-based health care: A JCN resource book for parish nurses,* 21–23.

This article details the development of a congregational health program initiated by Mercy Hospital in Pittsburgh and the process it used to reach out to various denominations within the inner city.

Boland, C. S. (1998). Parish nursing: Addressing the significance of social support and spirituality for sustained health-promoting behaviors in the elderly. *Journal of Holistic Nursing, 16 (3),* 355–368.

The importance of social support and spirituality to the empowerment of older adults to engage in health-promoting behaviors is a consistent research finding in this population. Parish nurse programs expand home health and public health provider roles by using the faith community as a means to implement successful health promotion programs.

Boss, J.G., and Yuen, T. (1995). Developing, implementing a cross-cultural lay health promoters program in an impoverished inner-city neighborhood. In National Parish Nurse Resource Center (Ed.), *Proceedings of Ninth Annual Granger Westberg Symposium,* pp. 135–149.

Buchheim, J. (1991). Rosalyn Grennan: Minister of health. *Church-based health care: A JCN resource book for parish nurses,* 30–33.

Buijs, R., and Olson, J. (2001). Parish nurses influencing determinants of health. *Journal of Community Health Nursing, 18 (1),* 13–23.

Carson, V. B. (2000). *Mental health nursing: The nurse-patient journey (2nd ed.).* Philadelphia: W. B. Saunders, p. 3.

———. (1989). *Spiritual dimensions of nursing practice.* Philadelphia: W. B. Saunders, pp. 55–56.

Chambers, O. (1993). *So I send you workmen of God.* Grand Rapids, MI: Discovery House Publishers.

In this small but powerful book Chambers enjoins all believers to reject the self-centered bent of a generation that seeks fulfillment in doing "what is best for me" and to find the fulfillment that God alone can give to his sons and daughters who in sacrifice and obedience seek His will above all else.

Chase-Ziolke, M. (1999). The meaning and experience of health ministry within the culture of a congregation with a parish nurse. *Journal of Transcultural Nursing, 10 (1),* 46–55.

This ethnographic study attempted to understand the meaning and experience of health ministry within a congregation. The author utilized participant observation, interviews, and reviews of written documents to develop an ethnography of an ethnically diverse, urban United Methodist congregation with a volunteer parish nurse. Two forms of health ministry were found within the congregation, which the investigator named extrinsic and intrinsic health ministry. Extrinsic ministry included activities whose explicit purpose was to promote health. Intrinsic health ministry included activities and experiences within congregational life whose express purpose was something other than health promotion, yet participants identified them as promoting their health.

————. (1997). Parish nurses help the elderly: The Northwestern Memorial Hospital Program. *Center on Aging, 13 (1)*, 4.

Chase-Ziolke, M., and Gruca, J. (2000). Client's perceptions of distinctive aspects in nursing care within a congregational setting. *Journal of Community Health Nursing, 17 (3)*, 171–183.

This qualitative research study described the client's experience of receiving nursing care within a congregation. Eleven individuals who utilized nursing services in two urban Catholic churches were interviewed. Content analysis revealed distinctive attributes experienced by participants in the relationship they had with the parish nurse. These included the manner of care, the focus of care, and the outcomes achieved. The ambience, time for interaction, and reflection of the connection between health and faith were seen as distinctive characteristics of the congregational setting.

Chase-Ziolke, M., and Striepe, J. (1999). A comparison of urban versus rural experiences of nurses volunteering to promote health in churches. *Public Health Nursing, 16 (4)*, 270–279.

These authors describe a research study comparing the practices of two parish nurse programs, one in a rural church and the other in an urban congregation. The two programs differed significantly regarding the location of the offered services. The nurses in the urban-based program provided most of their services at the church whereas the nurses in the rural-based program made many home visits and telephone calls in addition to the church-based services. Furthermore, the rural nurses were more involved in providing case management and practical interventions than their urban counterparts.

Clark, M. B., and Olson, J. K. (2000). *Nursing within a faith community: Promoting health in times of transition*. Thousand Oaks, CA: Sage Publications, Inc.

This book could be a textbook for a course in parish nursing. The authors represent two professional disciplines: nursing and theology. They use the knowledge bases of each of these disciplines to provide a truly interdisciplinary approach to this evolving model of nursing. They advocate for use of the terms "faith community" and "faith community nursing" rather than parish and parish nursing in order to extend the concept to the wide diversity of faith traditions existing throughout the world. The book is divided into seven sections: part I reflects on the similarities between faith seeking and health seeking; part II deals with theoretical foundations, developing conceptual foundations from both nursing and theological bases; part

III focuses on the role of the nurse as an agent of health promotion; part IV looks at promotion of health in times of transition; part V examines the process of nursing care within a faith community; part VI examines the role of faith communities in promoting images of health; and part VII examines the need to bring a vision of faith to bear on health and a vision of health to bear on faith.

Coenen, A., Weis, D. M., Schank, M. J., and Matheus, R. (1999). Describing parish nurse practice using the Nursing Minimum Data Set. *Public Health Nursing, 16 (6)*, 412–416.

Nineteen parish nurses practicing in twenty-two faith communities collected data using standardized nursing classification systems (North American Nursing Diagnosis Association Taxonomy [NANDA] and Nursing Intervention Classification [NIC]). A database was developed for quantitative analysis. Nurses recorded over 1,500 encounters for services provided to 776 individuals. Over the period of the study, nurses recorded 1,730 nursing diagnoses and 3,451 nursing interventions. The parish nurse roles that are reported in the literature were consistent with the findings of this study. The nurses also identified issues in using NANDA and NIC in documenting practice.

Conrad, D. (1995). Team nursing in parish nurse ministry: Even Jesus had 12 apostles. In National Parish Nurse Resource Center (Ed.), *Proceedings of Ninth Annual Granger Westberg Symposium*, pp. 105–110.

Cooney, R. (1994). Jerusalem, my destiny. In Robert J. Batastini and Michael A. Cymbala (Eds.), *Gather (2nd ed.)*. Chicago: GIA Publications, Inc.

Dahl, M. (Spring, 1994). Watch for G.M.C.'s, *Great is his love*. Moline, IL: Trinity Medical Center.

Deliganis, J. E. (1994). *Parish nurses' perceptions of their educational needs: A study of nurses who have attended the National Parish Nurse Resource Center's orientation program.* Unpublished doctoral dissertation, Texas A&M University, San Antonio.

Djupe, A. M., and Lloyd, R. C. (1992). Looking back: The parish nurse experience. National Nurse Resource Center.

Droege, T. (1995). Congregations as communities of health and healing. *Interpretation, 49 (2)*, 117–129.

Dunkle, R. M. (May 1996). Parish nurses help patients—Body and soul. *RN*, 55–57.

A small but growing number of nurses are providing wholistic care where a large number of Americans can be reached every week—at their church or synagogue.

Easton, K.L., and Andrews, J. C. (1999). Nursing the soul: A team approach. *Journal of Christian Nursing, 16 (3)*, 26–29.

Evans, C. (1995). The faith and public health partnership. *Our Connecting Point*, 1–2.

Fehring, R. J., and Frenn, M. (1987). Wholistic nursing care: A church and university join forces. *Church-based health care: A JCN resource book for parish nurses,* 24–27.

Ferngren, G. B. (1992). Early Christianity as a religion of healing. *Bulletin of the History of Medicine, 66,* 13–14.

Fowler, M. D. (1999). Relic or resource? The code for nurses. *American Journal of Nursing, 99 (3),* 56–58.

Freedman, M. (1999). *Prime time: How baby boomers will revolutionize retirement and transform America.* New York: Public Affairs.

Gaul, C. (June 21, 2001). If you ask them, they will come. *The Catholic Review, 67 (10),* 1, 3.

Gjerskvik, I. (1997). A heart of compassion: How nursing started in Norway. *Journal of Christian Nursing, 14 (2),* 12–13.

This article summarizes the efforts of Cathinka Guldberg, who was born on January 3, 1840 in Oslo, Norway, into a warm and loving Christian family. She often accompanied her father, who was minister, as he visited his congregation in rural areas. She learned at an early age the importance of charitable acts and she learned of the many unmet health needs that existed in her country. Cathinka traveled to Kaiserwerth, Germany, to receive her nurse's training and with that training returned to Norway to establish deaconness houses in Oslo. From Cathinka's early vision and commitment to God, deaconness nurses multiplied in Norway and today there are over 2,300 nurse graduates every year in Norway.

Greasley, P., Chiu, L. F., and Gartland, M. (March 2001). The concept of spiritual care in mental health nursing. *Journal of Advanced Nursing, 33 (5),* 629–637.

This study analyzed data from a series of focus groups to determine views of service users and mental health nursing professionals about the concept of spirituality and the provision of spiritual care in mental health nursing. The results indicated that spiritual care relates to an acknowledgment of a person's sense of meaning and purpose in life, which may or may not be related to formal religious beliefs and practices. The concept of spiritual care was also associated with the quality of interpersonal care in terms of the expression of care and compassion toward patients. However, concerns were expressed that the culture of mental health nursing was becoming less personal with increasing emphasis on the mechanics of nursing.

Griffin, J. (Spring/Summer, 2000). Personal perspective. *Perspectives in parish nursing practice.* Park Ridge, IL: Advocate Health Care, pp. 7–8.

Hall-Long, B. A. (1995). Nursing's past, present, and future political experiences. *N&HC: Perspectives on Community, 16 (1),* 24–28.

Contemporary public policy shifts and political opportunities make it important for the nursing profession to revisit the efforts of its political pioneers. Such historical inquiry can reveal "old truths about nursing's past and shed light on its emergence, helping to determine whether as a profession it has grown up or just grown older" in the public policy arena. In addition to reviewing some of nursing's political roots, an examination of nursing's policy research and political activities can offer insight to the profession for improved political transformations.

Hanson, C. M. (1991). The 1990s and beyond: Determining the need for community health and primary care nurses for rural populations. *The Journal of Rural Health, 7 (4),* 413–426.

Hatch, J., Moss, N., Saran, A., Presley-Cantrell, L., and Mallory, C. (1993). Community research: Partnership in black communities. *American Journal of Preventive Medicine, 9 (6),* 27–34.

Hatch, J.W., and Voorhost, S. (1992). The church as a resource for health promotion activities in the black community. In D. Becker, D. Hill, J. Jackson, D. M. Levine, F. Stillman, S. Weiss (Eds.), *Health behavior research in minority populations,* pp.30–34, (NIH Publication No. 92–2965). Bethesda, MD: U.S. Department of Health and Human Services.

Health Ministries Association and American Nurses Association. (1998). *Scope and standards of parish nursing practice.* Washington, DC: American Nurses Publishing, p. 1.

Holstrom, S. (1999). Perspectives on a suburban practice. In Phyllis Ann Solari-Twadell and Mary Ann McDermott (Eds.), *Parish nursing: Promoting whole person health within faith communities* (pp. 69–73). Thousand Oaks, CA: Sage Publications, Inc.

Hostutler, J., Kennedy, M. S., Mason, D., and Schorr, T. (2000). Nurses and models of practice. *American Journal of Nursing, 100 (2),* 82–83.

Since Florence Nightingale developed the foundations of modern nursing, nurses have continually created new models of practice that respond to changing times. Many of them reflect a desire for autonomy—the freedom to meet health needs in ways that deepen human caring, dignity, and well-being. The nurses profiled have worked toward that balance, inspiring us to act on our visions for nursing and health care.

Huggins, D. (1998). Parish nursing: A community-based outreach program of care. *Orthopedic Nursing* (March-April supplement), 26–30.

The goal is to help clients maintain the maximum level of wellness within their mental, intellectual, and physical capabilities.

Joel, L. A. (1998). Parish nursing: As old as faith communities. *American Journal of Nursing, 98 (8),* 7.

Kaplowitz, J. E. (1991). Community health advisors: A caring presence. *Journal of Christian Nursing, 8 (4),* 12–15.

This article describes the work of community health advisors who are trained by Christian nurses and educators of the Luke Society. These volunteers provide service under the direction of registered nurses and they work in some of the poorest communities in the United States. Although the service is not a parish nurse model, it includes one of the major components of the parish nurse role and that is to mobilize volunteers to meet the unmet health-care needs of a congregation.

Karaban, R. (1998). *Responding to God's call: A survival guide.* San Jose, CA: Resource Publications, Inc.

The concept of "call" is examined in this book. We are all called to be part of God's vision. We must recognize how God is calling each of us and how our piece of the vision fits into God's vision. Karaban states that the call to ministry begins as a story, a story of an encounter between an individual and God. This book presents a model for discerning God's call. Also examined is the close relationship between the discernment process and the grieving process. Frequently when God calls us, He calls us away from the familiar and into foreign territory. Responding always involves some loss as we give up our dreams to be replaced by what God dreams for us.

Kaufmann, M. A. (June 1997). Wellness for people 65 years and better. *Journal of Gerontological Nursing,* 7–9.

Keating, S. B. (1997). Parish nursing and home care. *Home Care Provider, 2 (5),* 204–205.

Kelleher, K. C. (1991). Free clinics—A solution that can work . . . now! *Journal of the American Medical Association, 266 (6),* 838–840.

Kelley, T. (2000). Reaching out to the unserved—Parish nurses fill void with a mix of physical and spiritual healing. *The New York Times,* pp. B1-B2.

King, J. M., Lakin, J. A., and Striepe, J. (1993). Coalition building between public health nurses and parish nurses. *Journal of Nursing Administration, 23 (2),* 27–31.

This article describes similarities between public health and parish nursing and discusses the nature of a collaborative relationship between these two groups of nurses.

Kiser, M., Boario, M., and Hilton, D. (1995). Transformation for health: A participatory empowerment education training model in the faith community. *Journal of Health Education, 26 (6),* 361–365.

The purpose of this article is to describe an application of participatory education methods in a hospital-based, community-oriented training project. It addresses one approach to a question now often asked, "How do professionals learn to value sharing power and decision making with individuals and the community?" By providing participatory, empowerment training, Mercy Hospital of Pittsburgh has demonstrated what is possible for health-care institutions seeking ways to develop effective partnerships with the community. At the same time, its actions identify a significant role the faith community can play in creating healthy communities.

Koenig, H. Presentation given March 4, 2001 at the "Faith in the future: Religion, aging, and healthcare in the 21st century" conference, Duke University, Durham, North Carolina.

Koenig, H. G., and Larson, D. B. (1998). Use of hospital services, religious attendance, and religious affiliation. *Southern Medical Journal, 91 (10),* 925–932.
Participation in and affiliation with a religious community is associated with lower use of hospital services by medically ill older adults, a population of high users of health-care services. Possible reasons for this association and its implications are discussed.

Koenig, H. G. (2002). *Purpose and power in retirement.* Philadelphia, PA: Templeton Foundation Press.

Koenig, H. G., McCullough, M. E., and Larson, D. B. (2001). *Handbook of religion and health.* New York: Oxford University Press, p. 29.

Kuhn, J. K. (1997). A profile of parish nurses. *Journal of Christian Nursing, 14 (1),* 26–28.

Lashley, M. E. (1999). Congregational care: Reaching out to the elderly. *Journal of Christian Nursing, 16 (3),* 14–16.

Lasseter, F. (1999). A nursing legacy: Political activities at the turn of the century. *AORN Journal, 70 (5),* 902, 904–907.
Nurses can look back on a rich history of political and professional achievements attained by their predecessors at the turn of the nineteenth century. The experiences and accomplishments of early nurses provide a strong foundation from which nurses today can enhance their profession and shape the public policy that affects it. The valiant efforts of America's nurse pioneers are best understood and appreciated in the context of the time. Nurses' early political involvement was the result of a variety of societal, economic, and political forces, and is inextricably linked with the introduction of formal education for women, the history of medicine, and the women's suffrage movement.

LeVasseur, J. (1998). Plato, Nightingale, and contemporary nursing. *Image–The Journal of Nursing Scholarship, 30 (3),* 281–285.
This article explores the influence of Plato's ideal of leadership on Nightingale's vision for nursing. Nightingale left her imprint on nursing; greater understanding of Nightingale's legacy clarifies several contemporary problems in the field.

Lloyd, R., and Djupe, A. M. (1993). Expanding our understanding of health and well being: The parish nurse program. Park Ridge, IL: Lutheran General Health System.

Lloyd, R., and Solari-Twadell, A. (1994). Organizational frame-work, functions, and educational preparation of parish nurses: National survey 1991–1994. In National Parish Nurse Resource Center (Ed.), *Proceedings of Eighth Annual Granger Westberg Symposium,* pp. 105–115.

Lough, M. A. (1999). An academic-community partnership: A model of service and education. *Journal of Community Health Nursing, 16 (3),* 137–149.

This article describes a unique clinical practice model in which an academic-community partnership was created between a college of nursing and a neighborhood grade school and parish. The partnership provided needed health services to patients, and at the same time gave students the opportunity to provide population-focused care in the community. The benefits of such a partnership include improved patient health status, increased access to health promotion services, and enhanced student learning.

Ludwig-Beymer, P., Welsh, C. M., and Tuzik-Micek, W. (1998). Keeping people healthy: Parish nursing's role in continuous quality improvement. *Journal of Christian Nursing, 15 (1),* 28–31.

Luks, A., and Payne, P. (1992). *The healing power of doing good.* New York: Ballantine Books.

Maddox, M. (2001). Circle of Christian caring: A model for parish nursing practice. *Journal of Christian Nursing, 18 (3),* 11–13.

Magilvy, J. K. and Brown, N. J. (1997). Parish nursing: Advanced practice nursing. Model for healthier communities. *Advanced Practice Nursing Quarterly, 2 (4),* 67–72.

These authors believe that the parish nurse model is an ideal model for the advanced practice nurse and allows the APN to contribute to healthier communities. The article goes on to describe models of parish nursing and the context and practice of the parish nurse with an emphasis on the issue of evaluating outcomes.

Marshall, J., Sorensen, E., Wall, R., and Mann, B. (1999). Religion, gender, and autonomy: A comparison of two religious women's groups in nursing and hospitals in the late nineteenth and early twentieth centuries. *Advances in Nursing Science, 22 (1),* 1–22.

This article compares cases of Catholic nuns and Mormon women as exemplars in a conceptual context of religious devotion, gender roles, and autonomy among women's religious organizations at the dawn of the twentieth century.

Martin, L. B. (January 1996). Parish nursing: Keeping body and soul together. *The Canadian Nurse,* 25–28.

Linda B. Martin (now Dr. Lynda W. Miller) discusses her own entry into parish nursing in Canada. She found a way to bring together her professional nursing experience as well as her spirituality as a member of a Christian faith community to devote herself to the whole person—spirit, soul, and body. She briefly reviews the evolution of parish nursing in the United States and in Canada and identifies issues that have an impact on the further development of this specialty within the Canadian health-care system.

Matheus, R. (Fall/Winter, 2000). Personal perspective. *Perspectives in parish nursing practice.* Park Ridge, IL: Advocate Health Care., pp. 6–7.

Matteson, M. A., Reilly, M., and Moseley, M. (2000). Needs assessment of home-bound elders in a parish church: Implications for parish nursing. *Geriatric Nursing, 21 (3),* 144–147.

The wholistic needs of elders in two parishes were determined through two multidimensional functional assessment questionnaires and a quality of life scale. Results indicate that this population of elders had relatively high levels of functioning. Quality of life was relatively high and was associated with overall functional abilities.

Matthews, D. A., Larson, D. B., and Barry, C. P. (1993). *The faith factor: An annotated bibliography of clinical research on spiritual subjects.* Rockville, MD: National Institute of Healthcare Research.

McConnel, C., and Zetzman, M. (1993). Urban/rural differences in health service utilization by elderly persons in the United States. *The Journal of Rural Health, 9 (4),* 270–279.

McCormick, P. (2001). Pass it on. *U.S. Catholic, 66 (8),* 46–48.

McDermott, M. A., and Burke, J. (1993). When the population is a congregation: The emerging role of the parish nurse. *Journal of Community Health Nursing, 10 (3),* 179–190.

McDermott, M. A., and Mullins, E. E. (1989). Profile of a young movement. *Church-based health care: A JCN resource book for parish nurses,* 4–5.

A survey gives demographic and employment data about thirty-seven nurses who work in churches.

McDermott, M. A., Solari-Twadell, P. A., and Matheus, R. (1998). Promoting quality education for the parish nurse and parish nurse coordinator. *Nursing and Health Care Perspectives, 19 (1),* 4–6.

In this article the authors provide a profile of the parish nurse as a professional who is involved in health promotion and disease prevention with spiritual care as the hallmark of the nurse's practice. In addition, the roles of the parish nurse are discussed, including health educator, health counselor, referral source, interpreter of the close relationship between health and faith, liaison with congregational and community resources, and facilitator and teacher of volunteers. Due to the growth and proliferation of parish nursing in the United States, Canada, Australia, and Korea (as of 1997), there is a need for standards for preparation and practice of parish nurses and their supervisors.

McElmurry, B., Wansley, R., Gugenheim, A., Gombe, S., and Dublin, P. (1997). The Chicago Health Corps: Strengthening communities through structured volunteer service. *Advanced Practice Nursing Quarterly, 2 (4),* 59–66.

McNamara, K. (Spring/Summer, 2000). Remembered forever. *Perspectives in parish nursing practice*. Park Ridge, IL: Advocate Health Care, p. 12.

Miles, L. (1997). Getting started: Parish nursing in a rural community. *Journal of Christian Nursing, 14 (1),* 22–25.

Miller, L. W. (1997). Nursing through the lens of faith: A conceptual model. *Journal of Christian Nursing, 14 (1),* 17–21.

In this article, Dr. Miller details the components of a wonderfully wholistic model: The Miller Model of Parish Nursing. In this model, developed for her doctoral dissertation, Dr. Miller identifies four major components: 1) person/parishioner, 2) health, 3) nurse/parish nurse, and 4) community/parish. These components are pictured in stained glass window designs. Within the center of this window are the core integrating concepts of the triune God, God's purposes, and personage. Around the periphery of the window are supporting concepts. Person/parishioner is supported by dignity and dependence; health is supported by the concepts of shalom-wholeness and stewardship; nurse/parish nurse is supported by mission and ministry; community/parish is supported by the concepts of confession and communion.

Morgan, L. (1999). Faith meets health: Religious congregation and outside agencies join together to promote public health. *Nurseweek (CA statewide ed.), 12 (17),* 8.

Morris, G. S. (1992). The Church Health Center and the Memphis Plan. *Health and Development, 12 (2),* 9–12.

Mustoe, K. J. (1998). The unbroken circle. *Health Progress, 79 (3),* 47–49.

Narayanasamy, A., and Owens, J. (February, 2001). A critical incident study of nurses' responses to the spiritual needs of their patients. *Journal of Advanced Nursing, 33 (4),* 446–455.

This study examined critical incidents to describe what nurses consider to be spiritual needs; explore how nurses respond to the spiritual needs of their patients; typify nurses' involvement in the spiritual dimensions of care; and describe the effects of nurses' interventions related to spiritual care. The study concluded that confusion exists about what exactly constitutes spiritual care and the nurse's role related to spiritual care. In addition, it was found that despite the lack of nursing consistency, spiritual care interventions promote a sense of well-being in nurses as well as being a valuable aspect of total patient care.

Nelson, B. J. (2000). Hospital extra. Parish nursing: Holistic care for the community. *American Journal of Nursing, 100 (5),* 24A–B, 24D.

The article discusses the role of the parish nurse in meeting the physical, emotional, psychological, and spiritual needs of the congregation and surrounding community.

Nelson, S. (1997). Pastoral care and moral government: Early nineteenth-century nursing and solutions to the Irish question. *Journal of Advanced Nursing, 26 (1),* 6–14.

This paper reexamines the role of the early nineteenth-century nurses, conventionally depicted in nursing histories as well-meaning but untrained Catholic nursing nuns or, in post-Reformation Europe, servants and fellow patients. It will be argued here that professional and capable nursing had begun to transform the care of the sick poor and to demonstrate its importance to the success of medical/surgical innovation long before Florence Nightingale and her call to Scutari. Moreover, the case is put that the emergence of nineteenth-century forms of care for the sick occurred in response to the pressing problems of population management in Ireland, Great Britain, and North America. The pastoral concerns of the first Irish nurses, with their expertise in both the spiritual and material domains, provided the prototype for what was to follow: a spiritual form of life that addressed the governmental concerns of its time. Finally, it is argued that given the overt moral imperatives of nineteenth-century nurses of all persuasions, the depiction of nursing history as a crossing from the religious to the secular domain is challenged.

Olson, J. K., Simington, J. A., and Clark, M. B. (1998). Educating parish nurses. *Canadian Nurse, 94 (8),* 40–44.

This article examines the growth of parish nursing in the United States as well as in Canada and the value of reconnecting nurses to their traditional roots in faith communities.

Oman, D., Thoresen, C., and McMahon, K. (1999). Volunteerism and mortality among the community-dwelling elderly. *Journal of Health Psychology, 4 (3),* 301–316.

Palmer, Jane. (First quarter, 2001). Parish nursing: Connecting faith and health. *Reflections on Nursing Leadership,* 17–19.

Parish nursing's pioneer: A JCN interview with Granger Westberg. *Church-based health care: A JCN resource book for parish nurses* (1989), 1–4.

Granger Westberg started several wholistic health centers, then decided nurses were the key. He shares the story behind parish nursing and how he became convinced that every congregation needs a parish nurse.

Parish nursing teaches prevention, wellness. *Patient Education Management, 4 (April 4, 1997),* 44–46.

This article focuses on the teaching and counseling roles performed by parish nurses. These functions are an invaluable tool to manage chronic diseases and reduce health-care costs.

Parker, M. (Summer, 2000). Mobilizing volunteers for service. *Healing Hearts and Hands, 4 (3),* 1.

Penner, S. J., and Galloway-Lee, B. (1997). Parish nursing: Opportunities in community health. *Home Care Provider, 2 (5),* 204–205.

This article addresses the changes in health care that have made community-based services, especially the role of parish nursing, so important in filling the gap in care. Specifically, the parish nurse lends support to the long-term care of those with chronic illnesses and promotes programs that provide health education.

Pisarcik-Lenehan, G. (1998). Free clinics and parish nursing offer unique rewards. *Journal of Emergency Nursing, 24 (1)*, 3–4.

Pruski, T. (August 10, 2000). Our congregations: Where physical and spiritual health can prevail. *The Catholic Standard*.

Quindlen, A. (2000). *A short guide to a happy life*. New York: Random House.

Remsen, J. (August 5, 2001). A pioneering Jewish "congregational" nurse offers holistic care: Ministering to the body and soul. *Philadelphia Inquirer*.

Ruesch, A. C., and Gilmore, G. D. (1999). Developing and implementing a healthy heart program for women in a parish setting. *Holistic Nursing Practice, 13 (4)*, 9–18.

The "Hearts to God" project was designed for implementation in a parish setting. The project integrates spirituality, stewardship, and wholeness into a cardiovascular health promotion program. The project includes exercises that enable women to assess, develop, and evaluate their own plan for heart health.

Russell, A. J. (1954). *God calling*. Uhrichsville, OH: Barbour Publishers.

This book provides daily devotionals to assist the seeker to hear and respond to God's call. In reading these devotionals a greater understanding of "call," "discernment," and "response" are possible.

Rydholm, L. (1997). Patient-focused care in parish nursing. *Holistic Nursing Practice, 11 (3)*, 47–60.

Rydholm examines the documented outcomes of parish nurse interventions and concludes that these interventions potentially result in Medicare cost savings. An analysis of 600 visits posits a $400,000 cost savings. Half of these estimates were related to scenarios where the caregiver was sustained to allow for ongoing home care. The other half were related to disregard of signs and symptoms warranting prompt attention. In both cases the interventions of advocacy, referral, assistance finding, active listening, and supportive education efforts were successful in removing stumbling blocks that prohibit access to care. By facilitating access, parish nurses ensured that earlier, simpler, more cost-effective treatment was made available rather than more complex and expensive care needed to treat conditions that were allowed to escalate.

Sabin, L. E. (1997). Charlotte of Aikens: An altered call. *Journal of Christian Nursing, 14 (2)*, 8–9.

Charlotte was born in 1868 in Mitchell, Ontario, Canada. She felt a call to missionary work and recognized the need to become a nurse so that she would be more fully prepared to serve in the missionary field. However, God led her in ways that did not include missionary work. Charlotte served as a nurse volunteer in the Spanish American War. After the war she served in many different leadership roles and contributed to nursing through prolific writings. She never served as a missionary but willingly responded to the Lord's leading. She wrote that there is no greater commendation for a nurse than to have been faithful to the Lord.

————. (1997). Claiming our heritage: Bridge to a lasting future. *Journal of Christian Nursing, 14 (2)*, 4–6.

In this article Sabin encourages today's nurse who may be discouraged by changes in the health-care system that devalue the caring aspect of nursing to find answers from the courageous nurses who established the profession of nursing many years ago. These nurses answered the call of God despite the fact that to do so meant a life of challenge and sometimes adversity. Today no less than yesterday we are still responding to the call of our God, who hears the cries of the poor and downtrodden and responds with compassion and care.

————. (1997). Fabiola: From arrogance to charity. *Journal of Christian Nursing, 14 (2)*, 7.

Sabin provides a brief history of Fabiola, born in the middle of the fourth century to a rich Roman family. Before her conversion to Christianity Fabiola was selfish, spoiled, and arrogant. After having married twice, Fabiola met Paula and Marcella, two wealthy Christian matrons living in Rome and studying the Scriptures with St. Jerome. Fabiola learned of Christianity and Christian charity from these mentors and committed her life to Christ after her second husband's death. She devoted her life to the sick and poor wherever she found them.

————. (1997). Hildegard of Bingen: A woman of vision. *Journal of Christian Nursing, 14 (2)*, 8–9.

Hildegard of Bingen lived in the twelfth century in central Germany. Hildegard was sickly and frail as a child and her family placed her with a noblewoman who had renounced the secular life to live as a contemplative recluse. Hildegard also responded to a call from God. She was a woman of vision who pursued many diverse avenues of service to God.

Salewski, R. (June 1993). Meeting holistic health needs through a religious organization: The congregation. *Journal of Holistic Nursing, 11 (2)*, 183–196.

This article discusses the comeback of Jesus' healing ministry in Christian congregations through the work of parish nursing. Parish nursing implements the gospel through health education, health counseling, patient advocacy, referrals, support groups, and the training of volunteers.

Schank, M. J., Weis, D., and Matheus, R. (1996). Parish nursing: Ministry of healing. *Geriatric Nursing, 17 (1)*, 11–13.

Parish nurses provide wholistic nursing services to members of church congregations.

Schank, M. J., Weis, D., and Matheus, R. (1996). Promoting well-being within a parish. *Canadian Nurse, 92 (1),* 20–24.

The implications of health reform for humanity are profoundly significant. It is important that reform results in healing and human fulfillment, not chaos and increased human pain. The parish and parish nurse have an important role in achieving positive health-care reform and returning much of the responsibility for health care to where it rightly belongs—the community.

Schlumpf, H. (2001). Call waiting: The stories of five women who want to be priests. *U.S. Catholic, 66 (2),* 13–17.

Schmidt, K. (1997). Victoria Schlintz: Answering God's call. *Journal of Christian Nursing, 14 (1),* 10–12.

Schmidt-Bunkers, S. (1998). A nursing theory—guided model of health ministry: human becoming in parish nursing. *Nursing Science Quarterly, 11 (1),* 7–8.

Schneider, E. L. (1999). Aging in the third millennium. *Science's Compass, 283,* 796–797.

Schumann, R. (1997). Documenting congregational nursing care: A model. *Journal of Christian Nursing, 14 (2),* 32–24.

Schumann describes a method of documenting the care provided by a congregational or parish nurse. The model includes a wholistic care summary noting personal information of the parishioner; summarizing the assessment of wholistic needs from an objective and subjective perspective; a follow-up evaluation that includes how many times the nurse met with the parishioner, number of times nurse contacted parishioner, success of referrals made by nurse; success of teaching/counseling as evidenced by change in parishioner's behavior; goals met or unmet; and modification of plan. In addition, the model includes a listing of short- and long-term goals, and planned wholistic care strategies that include teaching, counseling, referrals, advocacy within the congregation, and other strategies.

Schutte, D. (1994). Here I am, Lord. In Robert J. Batastini and Michael A. Cymbala (Eds.), *Gather (2nd ed.).* Chicago: GIA Publications, Inc.

Scott, L. (1992). *An adult and higher education perspective on the parish nursing experience.* Unpublished doctoral dissertation, University of South Dakota, Vermillion.

Scott, L., and Sumner, J. (1993). How do parish nurses help people? A research perspective. *Church-based health care: A Journal of Christian Nursing resource book for parish nurses,* 19–20.

Sensenig, J. (1993). *Nurse in the congregation: A guidebook for planning health ministries in Mennonite churches.* New Holland, PA: published by the author, p. 3.

Shelly, J. A. (2001). Parish nursing: Firing the imagination. An editorial. *Journal of Christian Nursing, 18 (3),* 3.

———. (Winter, 1997). Working toward shalom. *Journal of Christian Nursing, 14 (1),* 3.

Shelly, J. A., and Miller, A. B. (1999). *Called to care: A Christian theology of nursing.* Downers Grove, IL: Intervarsity Press.

This book examines the theological foundations for nursing. The content is organized around the nursing metaparadigm. Concepts such as the person, the environment, health, and nursing practice are explored from a biblical worldview. The authors also contrast this biblical worldview with modernism and postmodernism and demonstrate the impact that these competing worldviews are having on Christian nursing.

Sibbald, B. Hospital brings parish nursing to the community. *The Canadian Nurse, 98,* 22.

Interest in Canada's first acute care hospital-based parish nursing program is so great that Ottawa's Salvation Army Grace Hospital is launching a regional parish coalition.

Simington, R., Olson, J., and Douglass, L. (January 1996). Promoting well-being within a parish. *The Canadian Nurse,* 20–24.

Health reform is a social movement of profound human significance. Its impact will be felt by every person in our country. It is imperative that this movement result in healing and human fulfillment, not chaos and increased human pain. The first strategy for achieving positive health reform is to return much of the responsibility for health care to where it rightly belongs—the community. The second strategy is to develop more effective ways of fostering beneficial health behaviors in all persons.

Singer, N. (2001). Parish nursing: Jesus People style. *Journal of Christian Nursing, 18 (3),* 5–7.

Smith, S. D. (Spring, 1999). Response to God's life-giving ways by Ralph Underwood. *Insights, 14 (2),* 29–32.

Smith, S., Freeland, M., Heffler, S., McKusick, D., and the Health Expenditures Projection Team. (1998). The next ten years of health spending: What does the future hold? *Health Affairs, 17,* 128–140.

Smucker, C. J. (1989). Church nurse: Caring for a congregation. *Church-based health care: A JCN resource book for parish nurses,* 28–29.

Being a health minister means sharing both the highs and lows with people.

Solari-Twadell, P. A. (1997). The caring congregation: A healing place. *Journal of Christian Nursing, 14 (1),* 4–9.

Solari-Twadell, A. S. (Fall/Winter, 1999). Personal perspective. *Perspectives in parish nursing practice.* Park Ridge, IL: Advocate Health Care, pp. 7, 9.

Solari-Twadell, P. A. and McDermott, M. A. (1999). *Parish nursing: Promoting whole person health within faith communities.* Thousand Oaks, CA: Sage Publications.

This is an edited text representing a compilation of material from many authors involved in parish nursing. The book is divided into four sections: part I provides an overview of parish nursing as an emerging model of care; part II examines the role of collaborative practice as an essential component of parish nursing; part III looks at the context of practice for the parish nurse; part IV examines the challenges that exist for parish nursing as it expands across the world.

Solari-Twadell, A., and Westberg G. (1991). Body, mind, and soul. *Health Progress, 72 (7),* 24–28.

Solomon, L. (1989). Mobilizing an aids ministry in your church. *Church-based health care: A Journal of Christian Nursing resource book for parish nurses,* 34–36.

Souther, B. (1997). Congregational nurse practitioner: An idea whose time has come. *Journal of Christian Nursing, 14 (1),* 32–34.

Stewart, L. E. (May/June 2000). Parish nursing: Renewing a long tradition of caring. *Gastroenterology Nursing, 23 (3),* 116–120.
The author explores parish nursing as it is evolving into a model of nursing practice. This model contributes to the empowerment of the individual and the community.

Striepe, J. (1989). *Nurses in churches: A manual for developing parish nurse services and networks.* Park Ridge, IL: Parish Nurse Resource Center.

Striepe, J. M. (1993). Reclaiming the church's healing role. *Church-based health care: A A Journal of Christian Nursing resource book for parish nurses,* 6–9.

Striepe, J. M., and King, J. M. (1997). Basics for beginning a parish nurse program. *Church-based health care: A JCN resource book for parish nurses,* 14–17.

Striepe, J. M., King, J. M., and Scott, L. (1993). Nurses in the church: Profiles of caring. *Journal of Christian Nursing, 10 (1),* 8–11.

Stuchlak, P. (1992). Toning the temple: A church-based health fair. *Church-based health care: A JCN resource book for parish nurses,* 37–38.

Swinney, J., Anson-Wonkka, C., Maki, E., and Corneau, J. (January–February 2001). Community assessment: A church community and the parish nurse. *Public Health Nursing, 18 (1),* 40–44.
The results of an assessment of health needs of a parish in central Massachusetts is reported. A questionnaire along with focus group data were analyzed. The assessment was conducted by Amherst School of Nursing for a large urban parish. The assessment revealed that 93 percent of respondents felt they were in good health, 91 percent believed that faith and spiritual beliefs play an important role in health and well-being; and 70 percent believed that the church should play a role in helping parishioners meet their health needs. The focus group data revealed a need for respite care for primary care caregivers of the ill and elderly and educational programs for the teen and elderly populations.

U.S. Department of Health and Human Services (2001). *Healthy people 2010.* McLean, VA: International Medical Publishing.

Van Loon, A. (1998). The development of faith community nursing programs as a response to changing Australian health policy. *Health Education and Behavior, 25 (6)*, 790–799.

This article describes the faith community nursing roles (FCN) within Australia. The FCN demonstration project is described and the evolving FCN role and its relationship to the health-care continuum is discussed. Faith community nursing fosters not only community participation in health, but also whole person health within the specific context of a faith community.

Weber, C. (1994). Meeting holistic health needs through a religious organization: The congregation. *Beginnings, 14 (6)*, 1.

The healing ministry of Jesus is making a comeback in Christian congregations today through the parish nurse ministry. This ministry uses the wholistic health concept that health is an interplay of body, mind, and spirit. The parish nurse ministry implements the gospel message through health education and counseling, patient advocacy, referrals, support groups, and the training of volunteers.

Weiss, D. , Matheus, R., and Schank, M. J. (1997). Health care delivery in faith communities: The parish nurse model. *Public Health Nursing, 14 (6)*, 368–372.

This research study examined the monthly reports and parish nurse interviews and determined that parish nurse activities contributed to the empowerment process and to the attainment of *Healthy People 2000* objectives.

Wenger, A. F. (1992). Transcultural nursing and health care issues in urban and rural contexts. *Journal of Transcultural Nursing, 4 (2)*, 4–10.

Wessling, S. (1999). Nursing in a community of faith: The role of the parish nurse. *On-Call, 2 (4)*, 16–19.

This articles discusses the multitude of services provided by parish nurses whether working in paid or volunteer positions. These nurses improve the health of their communities by providing wholistic care, including the spiritual dimension.

Westberg, G. (1990). A historical perspective: Wholistic health and the parish nurse. In A. Solari-Twadell, A. M. Djupe, M. A. McDermott (Eds.), *Parish nursing: The emerging practice* (pp. 27–39). Park Ridge, IL: Lutheran General Health Care System.

————. (1990). *The parish nurse.* Minneapolis: Augsburg Fortress Press.

————. (1987). *The parish nurse: How to start a parish nurse program in your church.* Park Ridge, IL: Parish Nurse Resource Center, pp. 8–9.

————. (1986). The role of the congregation in preventive medicine. *Journal of Religion and Health, 25 (3)*, 1–4.

————. (1979). *Theological roots of wholistic health care.* Hinsdale, IL: Wholistic Health Centers.

Wilson, R. P. (1997). What does a parish nurse do? *Journal of Christian Nursing, 14 (1)*, 13–16.

Wurlitzer, F. P., and McIvor, A. C. (1996). Short term volunteer staffing of a hospital. *Southern Medical Journal, 89 (1),* 46–50.

Zarbock, S. F. (1997). Ministry of healing: a unique nursing role. *Home Care Provider, 2 (5),* 225–226, 228.

This article looks at one nurse's calling to become a parish nurse and examines the ministry that is available through the parish nurse role.

Zersen, D. (1994). Parish nursing: 20th-century fad? *Church-based health care: A JCN resource book for parish nurses,* 39–42.

Zetterlund. J. (1997). Kaiserwerth revisited: Putting the care back into health care. *Journal of Christian Nursing, 14 (2),* 10–11.

Zetterlund reviews the contribution made by Theodore and Friedericke Fliedner, considered the "father" and "mother" of deaconess nursing and other diaconal ministries within the Protestant tradition. Florence Nightingale received her nursing education at the Kaiserwerth, which was established with an understanding that Christ calls us to practice our faith through loving action toward others.

Index

professional development meetings, 101
Pruski, Tom, 68–72
Puget Sound Parish Nurse Ministries, 98, 101, 130

Quindlen, Anna, 85

research, faith and health, vii, 144, 145
resistance to parish nursing, 41
resources to start program, 125–27, 132

Schwartz, Morrie, 85
Scope and Standards of Parish Nursing Practice, xiv, 9, 138
Scott, Linda, 112–13, 128, 133
Sensenig, Joanne, 21, 97
Shelly, Rev. Jim, 129
Shelly, Judith, 35, 54, 125, 129, 140
Simmons, Dr. Harry, 103
Sisters of Mercy, 120
Small, Dr. Norma, 9, 95–96
Smith, Dianne, 18, 22, 33
Solari-Twadell, Ann, 11, 90–94
Spielman, Maggie, 76–79
spiritual gifts survey, 136
        STAR (Sexual Treatment, Advocacy, and Recovery) Center for Victims of Sexual Trauma, 80
steps for starting a parish nurse program, 124
Stoll, Dr. Ruth, 50, 96–98
Story, Carol, 98–102, 130
Stumpf, Terrill, 60, 81–83

support groups, 31
Swedish Covenant Hospital, 76
synagogue, congregational nurse, 111

Tavenner, Marilyn, 104
Teigen, Terry, 7, 30, 66, 72
Thomas, Rev. Sandra, 102–103
Thornton, Karen, 44, 59
Towers, Dr. Jan, 96
Trinity Medical Center, 17

Union Theological Seminary and Presbyterian School of Christian Education, 103, 144
University of Chicago, 87

volunteers, 2, 44
        training volunteers, 28, 29

Washington State Nurses Association, 100
Washington Theological Union, 95
Weinberg, Linda, 110
Wellness Works, 68
Westberg, Rev. Granger, vii, 12, 86–90, 143
Westberg Symposium on Parish Nursing, 91
"What to Do Until Help Arrives," 46
Whitesell, Linda, 46, 53
wholeness, 83
Wieringa, Joan, 30
worship, 82, 105–6

Young, Rose, 8